Practical Canine Behaviour

For Veterinary Nurses and Technicians

Practical Canine Behaviour

For Veterinary Nurses and Technicians

Stephanie Hedges

Certified Clinical Animal Behaviourist
Practising full member of the Association of Pet Behaviour Counsellors (APBC)
Registered Veterinary Nurse
APBC Veterinary Nursing representative
Lecturer in Companion Animal Behaviour and Therapy at Warwickshire College

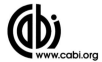

www.cabi.org

CABI is a trading name of CAB International

CABI	CABI
Nosworthy Way	38 Chauncy Street
Wallingford	Suite 1002
Oxfordshire OX10 8DE	Boston, MA 02111
UK	USA
Tel: +44 (0)1491 832111	Tel: +1 800 552 3083 (toll free)
Fax: +44 (0)1491 833508	Tel: +1 (0)617 395 4051
E-mail: info@cabi.org	E-mail: cabi-nao@cabi.org
Website: www.cabi.org	

A catalogue record for this book is available from the British Library, London, UK.

Library of Congress Cataloging-in-Publication Data

Hedges, Stephanie, author.
Practical canine behaviour: for veterinary nurses and technicians / Stephanie Hedges.
    p. ; cm.
  Includes bibliographical references and index.
  ISBN 978-1-78064-430-1 (pbk: alk. paper)
  I.C.A.B. International, publisher. II. Title.
  [DNLM: 1. Behaviour, Animal. 2. Dogs. 3. Animal Technicians. 4. Veterinary Medicine. SF 433]

SF433
636.7'0887--dc23

2014005541

ISBN-13: 978 1 78064 430 1

Commissioning editor: Julia Killick
Editorial assistant: Emma McCann
Production editor: Shankari Wilford

Typeset by SPi, Pondicherry, India
Printed and bound by Gutenberg Press Limited, Tarxien, Malta

Contents

About the Author

Stephanie entered veterinary practice as a student VN in 1990 and qualified as a Veterinary Nurse in 1992. She has worked in small animal general practice, orthopaedic and dental referral, and emergency and critical care practices, both in the private and charity sectors. She took an active and often lead role in training student nurses in practice and has also lectured on veterinary nursing, animal behaviour and animal care in both further and higher education in the UK.

Stephanie has always had an interest in canine behaviour, which developed further after adopting a GSD cross bitch from the RSPCA in 1999, who displayed a number of problem behaviours. This prompted her to study applied animal behaviour at the University of Southampton, graduating in 2004. She started to offer a limited in-house behavioural service at her practice in 2005, and established a part-time private referral service in 2006. Whilst taking referrals and working part time as a RVN she also completed a distance learning BSc (Hons) in Veterinary Nursing with Business Management, graduating in 2009 with a first.

Stephanie was accepted as a full member of the Association of Pet Behaviour Counsellors (APBC) in October 2009 and finally retired from nursing in November 2010. She now runs her own canine behavioural consultancy alongside lecturing undergraduates in companion animal behaviour at Warwickshire College, providing behavioural CPD to veterinary professionals and giving talks to trainers and the public. She also worked alongside other APBC members in training Local Authority Authorised Officers in the use of Dog Control Notices (DCNs) following the introduction of the Control of Dogs (Scotland) Act 2010 and as a consultant for the Guide Dogs for the Blind Association Breeding Centre.

In January 2012 Stephanie was invited to become the APBC's first Veterinary Nursing Representative and is now working with a team of other members to support UK VNs in practice by raising behavioural awareness and knowledge via a range of formats. She is also campaigning for the subject of behaviour to be included as a standard component of the VN syllabus.

She was accepted as a Certified Clinical Animal Behaviourist by the Association for the Study of Animal Behaviour (University of Nottingham) in 2013.

Preface

When I first started as a Veterinary Nurse I knew very little about canine behaviour. I had owned dogs and always loved dogs and felt I had a connection to them but there was so much I felt I did not know. After adopting Amber, a 1 year old female GSD cross, I came to learn so much more both through experience and formal study, whilst continuing to work as a nurse. As I did so it became apparent to me that understanding the natural behaviour of the animals we care for, learning how they communicate with us, appreciating the types of problems that can arise and perhaps most importantly how they can be prevented is a core aspect of a nurse's work. However the subject is still poorly reflected in the UK and US nursing syllabi.

There are many texts and courses available to develop the knowledge of both Veterinary Surgeons and Veterinary Nurses/Technicians hoping to specialize in behaviour, as I did. There are also books and courses aimed at enabling GP Veterinary Surgeons to address the medical aspects of behavioural issues before referral to a behaviour specialist. However, there is still little to address the needs to the GP VN/VT. This book aims to address this gap.

The book is divided into four sections. The first section covers the relevant principles of normal canine behaviour and communication, how normal and problem behaviour develops, how it can be changed and the human–canine bond. Understanding of these principles will help inform the later sections of the book, although are not essential for the time-strapped practitioner. The second section aims to highlight how advanced understanding of canine behaviour and communication can be used to improve handling and interaction with dogs in practice. The third section aims to summarize how the VN/VT can help prevent problem behaviour arising by offering appropriate advice and service to clients. The last section aims to guide VN/VTs how best to respond to clients presenting dogs with established problem behaviours. Guidance is given for those problems that can be addressed in the practice and flow charts are provided to guide when it is appropriate to refer to a specialist. This section also explains how to choose whom to refer to.

It is my hope that one day this level of understanding of behaviour will form an integral part of the Veterinary Nursing and Veterinary Technician syllabi. Hopefully, until then this book will go some way to offering help to nurses and technicians in everyday practice.

Acknowledgements

I genuinely could not have completed this book without the help and support of so many people.

First I must thank my army of proofreaders who provided so much useful feedback in their specialist areas and on general content and presentation. In alphabetical order these are Trudi Atkinson VN DipAS (CABC) CCAB, Gwen Bailey BSc (Hons), Sara Davies BVMS MRCVS DipCABT, Kris Glover BA (Hons) MSc (CABC) CCAB, Sophie Hacking BSc (Hons) MSc, Morag Heirs MSc MA (SocSci) (Hons) PGCAP, Elaine Henley PG Dip CABC, Chrissy Howell BSc (Hons) RVN, Michelle Smart RVN, Kate Smith BVSc MRCVS and Dr Hannah Wright BSc (Hons) PhD. Not forgetting the penguin posse of course, for filling in the gaps (you know who you are).

Next, but no less invaluable, are those who helped acquire the pictures and drawings. Top of this list has to be Laura Wyllie MAPDT of 'Laura Wyllie Dog Training' for her patient and steadfast help with this. That thanks automatically extends to all her friends, family, clients and dogs roped in as stooges and models. I would also like to thank White Cross Vets and Vets Now, both of Northampton, especially Sarah Rance RVN, for their help with the photos taken in practice. Extra photos were kindly supplied by Tom Worle of Tom Worle Photography, Graham Thompson, Joanne Drysdale, Sally Jones, Emma Brown and Natalie Light.

Finally, but of course most importantly, I would like to thank Amber, now sadly departed, for teaching me more than any book ever could, Rufus for making being a dog owner so easy – except when it comes to grass seeds! – and my son Jack for being there through the tears and the tantrums and always seeming to know when I need a cup of coffee – love you all.

Introduction

If an animal is physiologically ill or injured its suffering is obvious and need for veterinary treatment unquestioned. The threat to welfare of inappropriate behaviour is often less obvious. However, it has as much potential to impact negatively on a dog's quality of life as compromised physical health.

Where behaviour is normal and healthy for the animal but unwanted by the owner the dog may suffer loss of owner interaction or affection or, in more extreme cases, be at risk of physical punishment, abandonment or even euthanasia (see Box). Where the behaviour is driven by stress, fear, anxiety, frustration, conflict or depravation the threat to the dog's welfare is more direct and immediate. However, these states can often go unrecognized and the behaviour instead attributed to wilfulness, disobedience or traits such as being 'dominant' or 'aggressive'. Lack of recognition of the dog's true distress leaves them untreated or possibly punished, further compromising their welfare. As such, understanding, changing and preventing problem behaviour is as important to the dog's wellbeing as caring for his physical health.

Limitations of this text

The availability of companion animal training and behaviour services has mushroomed in recent years. This has brought with it an equally rapid growth in dedicated companion animal behaviour research. As knowledge has grown so has the need for practising companion animal trainers and behaviour specialists to undergo formal training and assessment. It is becoming widely accepted that this needs to be at undergraduate level for behaviour specialists, to enable the subject to be studied in sufficient depth and to develop the essential skills of diagnosis, treatment plan development and research evaluation. As such this text is insufficient on its own to equip the VN/VT as a behavioural specialist. The intention is that it will prepare the VN/VT for all behavioural matters relevant to their role in general veterinary practice and guide them when and where to refer on. It may also offer insight into a possible graduate or post-graduate course of study and career path for those with a specialist interest.

There are many areas in both psychology and animal behaviour that lack consensus, and many more that may require careful definition and discussion to appreciate properly. As this book is intended to be a guide for the practising nurse or technician I have avoided being drawn into these. That may mean academics will spot generalizations or simplifications. The intention is to make the text accessible and relevant to its target audience. It is no way meant to detract from the fascinating arguments that will no doubt for some time yet inform, challenge and delight the canine behaviour world.

To ease the flow of writing the text will use the male for personal pronouns. When doing so, reference is being made to either gender, except when specifically indicated.

The role of problem behaviour in rehoming and euthanasia of dogs.

- In a study of 5095 deceased dogs, 4% had been euthanized on behavioural grounds at a median age of 4.2 years old. Behavioural abnormality was the number one reason for euthanasia in dogs under 3 years of age (O' Neill *et al.*, 2013).
- Behaviour problems are the number one cause of relinquishment to shelters in the USA (Miller *et. al.*, 1996; Salman *et al.*, 1998).
- Up to 89% of dogs returned to rescue charities are returned due to a behavioural problem (Wells and Hepper, 2000).
- Dogs euthanized by rescue shelters are predominantly destroyed on behavioural grounds (Bollen and Horowitz, 2008).
- Dogs euthanized on behavioural grounds are on average much younger (median lifespan 4 years compared to overall median lifespan of 13 years) (Stead, 1982; Mader and Hart, 1992).

PART 1
Principles of Behaviour

Introduction

The principal aim of this book is to provide practical advice on improving the behavioural management of dogs both within the practice and at home. However, application of this advice can be informed and so improved with theoretical understanding of the key principles of canine behaviour. Many may also like to further their understanding of canine behaviour, for its own sake. The first section of the book will therefore provide an introduction to key aspects of canine behaviour and its modification. It will not be sufficient to prepare practice staff to act as specialist behavioural advisers. However, it will offer an insight into the influences over canine behaviour and ways in which it can be manipulated.

1   The Human–Animal Bond

The behaviour of a pet dog is inextricably linked with that of his owner. As such, the owner's needs, expectations, perception of their dog's behaviour and reasons for keeping the dog always need to be considered and understood when looking to manage the dog's behaviour.

Why Do People Keep Dogs?

Looked at superficially, keeping a dog can sometimes seem like an act of altruism. An owner must sacrifice time and resources to keep the animal, often without any apparent reciprocation. However, if we look a little deeper it can be seen that dogs fulfil many beneficial roles in human lives. These are summarized in Table 1.

Human Attitudes to Animals

Human attitudes towards animals in general and dogs in particular vary widely. This applies equally to the owner and to others affected by the dog such as family, neighbours and wider society.

Attitudes can be influenced by upbringing, experience, psychological and emotional development and personal circumstances. Religion, culture and relative affluence also have a bearing on an individual's attitude. For example some religions forbid keeping of certain pets, whereas others may recognize the spirituality of pets and some people may extend their religious beliefs to them. Those having greater wealth are better able and so more likely to provide for companion animals or see it as acceptable to do so.

Owner perception of their relationship with their dog

The way in which a person perceives their relationship with their dog will affect their expectations and perception of their pet's behaviour. Types of relationship are discussed in Table 2.

Anthropomorphism

Anthropomorphism is the attribution of human characteristics to non-human beings, objects or abstract concepts. Humans are often guilty of anthropomorphizing their dogs. However, the degree to which they are maligned for doing so may be unfair.

As we can never truly know what another is feeling or the triggers for their behaviour we use empathy to interpret it. This applies equally to humans and other species. The only way we can understand behaviour is as a human. It is therefore natural our interpretation of a dog's behaviour will be from a human perspective. The domestication of the dog, and some argue the evolution of the human, has led to many similarities in the social and emotional behaviour of the two species. Our anthropomorphic interpretation may therefore sometimes be correct. However, care must be taken to recognize differences between human and canine drives, methods of communication, emotions and intellectual abilities. Assuming and responding as if a dog's behaviour is wholly the same as human's carries great risk and is often the reason for problems in behaviour or the dog:human relationship. A balance therefore has to be struck. The influences over dog behaviour are discussed further in Chapters 2–4.

Dissociation

Dissociation is the psychological process by which humans emotionally distance themselves from an individual animal or species of animal. This is normally reserved for species kept for utilitarian purposes such as food or work. However, some owners may also do so with their pets. For example they may use dissociation as a protective mechanism if they fear emotional distress as a result of becoming attached to the dog, perhaps due to experience. They may alternatively use it as a psychological coping mechanism if they are forced to make a difficult decision regarding the pet, e.g. to have a dog that has bitten euthanized under court order.

Table 1. Reasons for keeping dogs.

Beneficial role	Discussion
Companionship	The principal reason for keeping dogs in western society is companionship and emotional fulfilment, instead of or alongside human relationships. However, the degree of emotional attachment and commitment to the dog, ranging from integral family member to disposable possession, may vary widely between individuals, even within the same family.
Amusement	Dogs may be kept for sport or hobbies, e.g. showing or competition. If they do not fulfil this niche they may then be disposed of.
Image	People may keep certain breeds to project a desired image. This may include to suggest menace, power, individuality or to publicly associate with others, e.g. celebrities.
Social facilitation	Dogs can be kept to provide an opportunity or motivation for interaction with other humans.
Child development	Dogs play a beneficial role in child development, teaching them about caring for another, responsibility, reproduction and death. Pet keeping is also known to teach empathy and promote the child's self-esteem, cognition and emotional functioning.
Health	Owning a dog can promote exercise. It has also been demonstrated to improve health through reductions in blood pressure and ailments associated with chronic stress.
Utility	Utilitarian roles may include assistance dogs, guard dogs, rodent control, herding, hunting or financial reward, e.g. breeding, racing.

Table 2. Types of dog–human relationship.

Perceived relationship	Discussion
Ownership	Most people perceive their dog as theirs to own and control. Ownership brings both rights and responsibilities. An owner has a right to determine the basis of their relationship as long as it does not compromise the welfare of the dog. However, they also have a moral and legal responsibility to provide for the dog's needs and to ensure he does not infringe the rights of others by being a nuisance. A few may see the dog as a free spirit who makes his own decisions. They therefore do not feel they have to take responsibility for him or what he does.
Symbiosis	Relationships can be mutualistic, commensal or parasitic. Which of these categories any given dog–human relationship falls into can vary, but is ultimately determined by the human. Each individual's perception of the balance between fulfilment of their own, others and the dog's needs will vary according to their attitude to or importance attached to their dog.
Transference	An owner may choose a dog, or have expectations regarding their dog's behaviour, that reflect their own (perceived) traits. For example, a very self-disciplined person may expect their dog to be very well behaved too.
Superimposition	An owner may interpret a dog's behaviour in a way that reflects what the owner thinks or wants the animal to show, rather than the actual behaviour being performed or motivation behind it. For example if a dog shows aggression to a stranger in the street the owner may believe the dog is trying to protect them, which makes them feel cared for, when in fact the dog is trying to protect himself.
Release	An owner may like the dog to perform things they are unable to, whether perceived or in reality. An example may be a self-disciplined person who finds release in the lack of discipline their dog shows.

2   What Influences Behaviour

Before looking specifically at the behaviour of the dog it is useful to appreciate the many factors that influence behaviour. For simplicity, behavioural influences can be broadly placed into three categories, i.e. nature, nurture and the current environment.

Nature includes the anatomical and physiological controls that determine and regulate normal behaviour and the pathological processes that may disturb it. Nurture describes all the influences that affect a dog's development and learning. The current environment reflects triggers and stimuli affecting the dog at any given time and the behaviour of others around him.

Nature

All behaviour is at least partly influenced by and is under the ultimate control of an individual's anatomy and physiology. There are numerous physiological drives to perform particular behaviours and whatever the dog's past experiences and current situation, he can only perform those behaviours to which he has the physical ability. These influences must therefore be fully understood and considered when attempting to understand or modify a dog's behaviour.

Genetic inheritance

Genes are molecular units that hold the code for building proteins, which in turn determine the structure and govern the function of an organism's cells. Each species has its own genomic sequence, within which there will be individual variation. As such, genetically driven behaviours tend to be similar within species, but show some variation between individuals or subsets of individuals, e.g. breeds. This variation is influenced by a number of factors, summarized in Table 3.

Evolution

For an animal to survive its behaviour must be 'adaptive', i.e. the behaviour must maximize the species' chances of surviving and reproducing and so passing its genes into the next generation. In more advanced species this also includes more complex behaviours. For example the success of a social species relies on interactions between group members. The animal's social behaviour therefore has to be adaptive for it to survive.

The behaviour of most individuals within a species will be the one that gives the best chance of survival and reproduction. 'Survival of the fittest' refers to survival of the 'most fit'. However, the genetic influences discussed above mean that there will always be some variation. If a variation is slight or does not have a behavioural consequence the individual carrying it may still survive and reproduce and so may pass that gene on to the next generation. However, more extreme variations may interfere with the ability to function normally and so are less likely to be passed on. Even minor variations may also be weeded out when there is strong competition for limited resources.

Behaviour will evolve – i.e. change in the majority of the population – when something causes a change to the most adaptive behaviour. That may be a change in the climate, the animal's environment or a change in the behaviour of other species that compete for the same resources. Some genetic variations can then start to be advantageous, increasing the likelihood those carrying them will survive and eventually become the most common.

In short, evolution will ensure most individuals within a species behave in the most adaptive way for their current environment. However, there will always be some variation, and if the animal's environment changes then their behaviour will also gradually change to suit it. The environmental changes

Table 3. Factors influencing genetic and phenotypic variation between individuals.

Influence	Discussion
Gene combination	Two alleles are inherited for each gene. Ordinarily only one influences structure or function, i.e. is dominant. However, some alleles may be co-dominant, meaning both are demonstrated, and some may be incompletely dominant meaning they are only weakly demonstrated. Some genes may have multiple alleles and so potential influences (polymorphs), some are linked so are always displayed together, some genes have multiple influences (pleiotrophy) and the intensity of gene demonstration may vary where multiple genes have the same effect (e.g. hair colour). As such, each animal's phenotype will depend on the specific and complex combination of its genes.
Gene mutation	A gene may reproduce incorrectly and so change at any division after conception. This then affects the structure and function of future cells.
Epigenetics	Gene expression can be switched on or off by factors such as environment, diet and stress.

that are most likely to have affected the evolution of the dog are discussed in Chapter 3.

The endocrine system and hormones

Hormones are chemical messengers. They are produced by cells or glands in one part of the body and then travel via the vascular system to affect the functioning of cells in other parts of the body. As hormones affect physiology they will all affect behaviour to some degree.

Stress hormones

Stress is the body's physiological and/or behavioural response when adverse environmental conditions 'over-tax' the individual's adaptive coping mechanisms. This definition reflects that many environmental stimuli may be adverse but can often be adapted to through normal homeostatic functions. It is only when normal coping mechanisms cannot fully rectify the adverse stimulus that stress responses occur. For example, extreme heat may be adverse but its effects can normally be regulated by temperature control mechanisms such as panting. Stress therefore only occurs when the adverse effects of heat cannot be corrected in this way, causing elevation in core body temperature.

Stress may be acute or chronic. Acute stress is short lived and occurs as the initial response to an adverse stimulus. The physiological process of acute stress is discussed in Box 2.1. These physiological changes are designed to increase the individual's cognitive and physical ability to respond to acute stress by defending itself (fight) or escaping (flight). As these hormones are designed to respond to acute stress they have a rapid effect. However, once circulating levels reach a given level they will trigger a negative

feedback mechanism that inhibits long term production. They are therefore short lived.

Chronic exposure to stressful stimuli triggers longer term adaptive responses through the hypothalamic pituitary adrenal (HPA) axis. The physiological process of chronic stress is discussed in Box 2.2. Elevated levels of blood cortisol are intended to enable the body to return to normal homeostasis after acute stress or to cope with on-going external stressors. Its effects are therefore adaptive and at normal levels are possibly even desirable. On-going cortisol levels are regulated through stimulation of a negative feedback mechanism once corticotrophin-releasing hormone (CRH) and adrenocorticotrophic hormone (ACTH) thresholds are reached. However, if external stressors are extreme, recurrent or protracted they can interfere with normal cortisol regulation mechanisms. This may lead to excessive responses or maladaptive coping behaviours.

Other hormones may also play a part in the regulation of stress. Some may have a role in the synthesis, metabolism or potentiation of principal behavioural hormones or minor effects in processes primarily regulated by the hormones discussed above. They may also have indirect effects, such as glucagon and insulin regulation of energy levels impacting on the ability to maintain homeostasis. The roles of most of these hormones only become truly behaviourally relevant when they are disrupted due to disease. This is discussed further below.

Endocrine influences on sexual dimorphism

At conception the zygote is genetically either male or female. However, the physiological and behavioural differences between the sexes, referred to as

Box 2.1. Physiological effects of acute stress.

- Acute stress triggers the sympathetic aspect of the autonomic nervous system to release the catecholamines epinephrine and norepinephrine.
- This results in increased glucose and oxygen delivery to vital organs through:
  - Tachycardia
  - Tachypnoea
  - Increased cardiac output
- Bronchial dilation
- Vital organ vasodilation with peripheral vasoconstriction
- Glycolysis and glycogenolysis.
- The result is increased strength, endurance and cognitive ability to augment the 'fight' or 'flight' response.

Box 2.2. Physiological effects of chronic stress.

- CRH is produced in the anterior aspect of the paraventricular nuclei in the hypothalamus and conveyed by portal circulation to the corticotrophs in the anterior pituitary.
- Here it stimulates production of ACTH, which in turn releases the glucocorticoid cortisol from the adrenal gland cortex.
- The metabolic effects of raised blood cortisol include:
  - Elevated amino acid concentration due to reduced muscle protein synthesis and increased muscle protein catabolism
- Hyperglycaemia due to increased lipolysis and inhibition of glucose uptake in the cells
- Interference with normal immune and inflammatory responses
- Interference with memory formation
- Hypertension
- Long-term elevated blood cortisol can lead to muscle wastage and weight loss.

sexual dimorphism, arise due to a combination of genetic gender and the influence of hormones during development.

If the embryo is genetically male a gene code found only on the Y chromosome will trigger testosterone production at various intervals through gestation and just prior to parturition. This will have a masculinizing effect on the pituitary gland, which will in turn trigger the embryo to develop male gonads, a heightened sensitivity to testosterone and male patterns of behaviour after birth. The lack of this influence in female embryos leads to the development of female gonads, heightened sensitivity to oestrogen and female behaviour patterns. These effects are unaffected by neutering.

As the dog reaches puberty there will be further surges in testosterone and oestrogen, which will have further influence over brain organization. This is again unchanged after subsequent neutering.

Because gender-specific physiology and behaviour relies on a combination of genetics and hormonal influences, variation can occur. For example, where a genetically male brain receives a lower than usual 'wash' of testosterone the embryo may fail to develop male genitalia, masculine characteristics such as body mass, male behaviour patterns or male typical sensitivity to testosterone. How marked this is depends on to what degree the testosterone is reduced and the stage of development affected. This is known to occur in males from dams that are stressed perinatally due to the suppressive effects of cortisol on testosterone.

Alternatively, if a female embryo receives a testosterone wash, perhaps triggered by male siblings *in utero*, she may develop sensitivity to testosterone. This is referred to as androgenization. Although she will still ordinarily have much lower levels of circulating testosterone, this will have a greater effect than normal on behaviour if she sensitized in this way. Affected females may show leg cocking, increased aggressive behaviour and disrupted seasonal cycles.

Endocrine influences on sexual behaviour

Reproductive drive and sexual competition in the male is regulated by testosterone. Castration removes the principal site of production for testosterone and so reduces such drives. However, if performed after behaviours have become established they may persist due to learning or habit formation.

Testosterone produced in the adrenal cortex is generally considered insignificant in entire dogs. However, it may become more so once gonads are removed and so neutering may not entirely remove reproductive drives in all cases.

The hormonal control of female reproductive behaviour and sexual competition is more complex. The key hormones and their roles are summarized in Table 4.

Endocrine influences on aggression

Testosterone increases production of noradrenaline and arginine vasopressin (AVP also known as ADH), which in turn increase arousal and approach, and the speed, intensity and duration of aggressive responses. Testosterone also increases risk-taking behaviour,

reduces fear (van Honk *et al.*, 2005) and is thought to be linked to the sensations of reward. There is a complex interaction between the stress hormone cortisol and testosterone. Testosterone levels are typically, although not consistently, reduced by cortisol. However, testosterone also has the ability to inhibit the HPA axis stress response, depending on circumstances.

The nervous system

The nervous system controls sensory input and motor actions. As such, physiology has a key role to play in how information is received and responded to.

The anatomy and categorization of the structures in the brain is complex, at times contentious and continually changes to reflect new findings. Knowledge of this is not essential for understanding the

Table 4. Female hormones and their effect on sexual behaviour.

Hormone	Role
Follicle stimulating hormone (FSH)	Produced by the anterior pituitary gland. Triggers development of Graafian follicles and testosterone production (in the female). Raised levels occur post-neutering.
Oestradiol	Produced by Graafian follicles, causing swelling of the vulva, vulval discharge and attractiveness to males.
Oestrogen	Produced by the maturing Graafian follicle. Gradually increases over 4–5 weeks, supressing FSH and LH, then suddenly drops enabling a luteinizing hormone surge and ovulation. Causes increased activity, marking, vocalization and arousal. Lowers the threshold for (so increases the incidence of) aggression, facilitating sexual competition with other females and keeping males away until ready to be mated.
Luteinizing hormone (LH)	Produced by the anterior pituitary. Starts at the same time as FSH but levels are kept low by oestrogen. Surges when oestrogen levels drop, triggering ovulation and resulting corpus luteum.
Progesterone	Produced by the corpus luteum for around 55 days post-ovulation, whether pregnant or not, although is marginally lower in non-pregnant bitches. Increases the threshold for (i.e. reduces the incidence of) aggression, so the male is accepted. Calms the dam and maintains the pregnancy. Falls in late pregnancy/metoestrus.
Prolactin	Produced by the pituitary. Rises as progesterone starts to fall, whether pregnant or not. Triggers mammary enlargement and milk production, nesting, mothering and protective aggression. Prepares for parturition in the pregnant bitch, or may trigger a pseudopregnancy if not. The intensity of physical and behavioural signs of pseudopregnancy can vary. Sudden behavioural changes such as onset of aggression may occur even where more obvious signs of pseudopregnancy are silent.
Oxytocin	Produced by the posterior pituitary. Triggers contractions during parturition, release of milk in response to touch stimulation of nipples, maternal behaviour and bonding between dam and puppies.
Testosterone	Produced by the thecal cells in the ovaries, the placenta and the adrenal cortex. Most (but not all) ovarian testosterone is converted to oestrogen. However, testosterone levels rise in pro-oestrous and can be as high as males by the time of the LH surge (Olsen *et al.*, 1984).

influence of the nervous system on behaviour. This section will therefore only consider the behavioural effects of central nervous system activity.

Neurological influences on learning, memory and emotion

Learning, memory and emotion are closely linked. Learning is of little use without effective memory formation and retrieval. Memory influences learning by placing it in the context of past experience and enables the learning to be applied in subsequent situations. For example, for a dog to learn that barking for attention does not work then he may need to try and fail a number of times. This requires memory. Trying something new (e.g. sitting for attention) also requires recollection of what has been tried before.

Emotion also affects memory formation and learning. Intensely emotional experiences are often remembered much more clearly than non-emotional events. Mild anxiety may facilitate learning, but intense fear may interfere with some forms of learning as the drive for survival takes precedence. Learning is discussed more in Chapter 7.

Neurological influences on fear and aggression

Aggression in animals can be predatory or affective. Predatory aggression is controlled by the lateral hypothalamus and triggers similar reward sensations as eating and drinking. Affective aggression describes aggressive behaviour used in defence or to protect something of value. It is regulated by the medial hypothalamus, periaqueductal grey matter (PAG) and amygdala, among other structures. The PAG is linked to sensations of anxiety, distress, panic and terror. The amygdala is linked to fear, anxiety and emotional learning. It can therefore be seen that the emotional effects of these two types of aggression are opposing. This is discussed further in Chapter 6.

Neurotransmitters

Neurotransmitters are endogenous chemicals that regulate the transmission of nerve impulses. They are produced in the nerve body and stored in the presynaptic axon terminal buttons. If the neuron is activated the impulse causes release of the neurotransmitter into the synaptic cleft where it then attaches to receptors on the dendrites of the post synaptic cell.

Neurotransmitters can be excitatory (increase the chance of activation), inhibitory (decrease the chance of activation) or have the potential to be either, dependent on the receptor with which they dock. The type and quantity of neurotransmitters released will vary, as will the type and number of receptors available to attach to. The activity of the next cell is therefore determined by the combination of which neurotransmitters are released, in what quantity and to which receptors they attach.

After the neurotransmitter has docked and activated the receptor it is then released back into the synaptic cleft. It may then reattach to further influence the activity of the post-synaptic cell, may be broken down or may be reabsorbed back into the terminal button. The neurotransmitters most relevant to behaviour modulation are summarized in Table 5. The specialization of the canine senses is discussed in Chapter 5.

Body rhythms

Circadian rhythms

Circadian rhythms are behavioural cycles that vary with the time of day. Each species will have periods of high and low activity, coupled with associated or regulatory physiological changes, determined by the time of day to which they are most adapted. Examples of physiological changes include a reduction in body temperature during the animal's normal sleep phase and increased urine production during normal waking periods, regardless of whether the animal is actually awake or asleep at that time. The circadian biological clock works independently of external cues. However, it is 'set' daily, to ensure it does not deviate too far from the 24 h cycle and that it reflects the local periods of day and night. It will be reset if these are disrupted (e.g. when the clocks change) although there will be a period of transition that may cause distress. Dogs are crepuscular and so most active at dawn and dusk.

Breeding cycles

Each species undergoes different cycles of fertility and associated receptivity to mating. In the dog these cycles are hormonally controlled. The behaviour of the dam undergoes substantial changes over the duration of her cycle. The behaviour of the sire

Table 5. Neurotransmitters relevant to behaviour modulation.

Neurotransmitter	Activity
Serotonin	Elevated mood and regulation of sleep cycles. Reduced levels are linked to aggression and stress.
Norepinephrine	Is synthesized from dopamine. May be excitatory or inhibitory. Increases heart and respiratory rate in emergencies. Heightens mood and arousal, and increases reward and attention.
Epinephrine	Excitatory. Short-acting response to danger or acute stress. Increases cardiac and respiratory function.
Dopamine	Excitatory. Increases motivation, confidence, exploration, attention, approach and pleasure from rewards. Reduces apprehension. Improves problem solving and learning, including responses to training.
Gamma-aminobutyrate acid (GABA)	Inhibitory. Prevents neurons firing in response to other neurotransmitters. Reduces fear and anxiety.
Glutamate	Excitatory. Inhibited by GABA. Influential in learning and memory.
Acetylcholine	May be excitatory or inhibitory, depending on the receptor. Affects memory, arousal, attention and mood.

can also be affected if there are bitches in heat in their vicinity.

Diet

An animal's nutritional status can affect behaviour in many ways. General malnutrition, obesity or an excess or deficit of one or more specific nutrients may interfere with physiological function. The increased tendency towards home-made diet adds to the risk of dietary imbalance or malnourishment. Feeding a poor quality or unsuitable commercial diet may also lead to problems. For example, prolonged use of puppy diets or feeding a working dog food to a family pet can give the dog higher energy than is required resulting in excessive activity and irritability. Some also suggest certain ingredients can adversely affect behaviour above and beyond dietary sensitivity. However, there is so far no formal research to support this.

Blood sugar fluctuations

Feeding infrequently or diets high in sugar may lead to fluctuations in blood sugar levels. High blood sugar can cause increased irritability or arousal. Low blood sugar can lead to increased value placed on resources and competition for food.

Protein/carbohydrate balance

There is evidence to suggest that heightened aggression or arousal may be seen in dogs fed a high protein diet. This is thought to be due to the increased circulating levels of tyrosine and phenylalanine, as precursors to catecholamines, or competition between tryptophan hydroxylase (THP) and large neutral amino acids (LNAA) derived from dietary protein.

THP plays a significant role in the anabolism of serotonin (5-HT), a monoamine neurotransmitter responsible for gut regulation, cardiovascular function, growth and central nervous system (CNS) regulation of mood, appetite, sleep, memory and learning. 5-HT is produced in the gut and the raphe nuclei in the brainstem. However, 5-HT produced in the gut or taken orally cannot cross the blood–brain barrier (BBB). It is therefore essential that sufficient THP is able to enter the CNS to enable brainstem metabolism of 5-HT. THP uses the same transporter mechanism as some other LNAAs to cross the blood–brain barrier, so they are in competition. As such, increased circulating LNAAs from the diet will decrease the quantity of THP crossing the blood–brain barrier and so levels of serotonin in the brain.

Potential effects of additives

Recent research has lent scientific support to claims that certain food colours can impact on the behaviour of some children (McCann et al., 2007). The additives implicated are summarized in Box 2.3. A label highlighting their potential effect on the behaviour of children is now required on foods containing them in the UK and some other countries.

Some dog foods contain the implicated additives although to date there is no evidence to support or refute the potential effects of these additives on canine behaviour. Anecdotal reports suggest beneficial changes in behaviour following a change to a diet free of these additives. However, any changes seen following a change of diet may arise due to many factors, including other concurrent behaviour modification steps taken and the tendency for diets high in additives to have poorer nutritional value and/or be higher in sugar. The true cause of any changes seen is therefore not yet established.

Illness and injury

Any illness can affect behaviour. The behavioural implications of generic clinical signs seen in many conditions are summarized in Table 6.

In many cases there will be physical clinical signs alongside the behavioural ones, so the role of disease in development of the behaviour will be clear.

However, in some cases the behaviour changes may be the first indication of an otherwise subclinical condition. Where a dog's behaviour genuinely changes suddenly or is 'out of character', especially at a time of life when the dog is not expected to be undergoing behavioural changes, the likelihood it is due to disease is increased. Behaviour that is inconsistent or incongruous with triggers also has a higher likelihood of a physical influence.

Where the likelihood of a physical cause for behavioural signs is unclear the veterinary surgeon will need to decide whether to perform further diagnostic tests or make a referral. Asking the client to keep a behavioural diary or make a video recording of behaviour can often help determine the right course of action. Referral to a qualified behavioural specialist can also form part of the diagnostic work-up by identifying or eliminating purely behavioural causes for the clinical signs being displayed. In some cases this may be the more economical option, depending on the nature of the alternative tests indicated.

Pain

Physical pain is typically triggered by strong mechanical stimulation that stretches, bends or damages the pain receptors, known as nociceptors. It may also be caused by extremes of temperature, oxygen deprivation or the effects of certain chemicals. If any of these triggers results in tissue damage the pain will be protracted. The nature and intensity of

Table 6. Behavioural effects of generic clinical signs of illness or injury.

Clinical sign	Discussion
Disruption to the normal function of anatomy	Interference with movement will change the dog's behavioural responses in trigger situations, e.g. force fight instead of flight. Prevention of coping mechanisms may increase anxiety. Loss of sensory input will affect perception or reaction to situations and increase anxiety or sense of vulnerability. Illness or injury may also interfere with normal communication.
Polyuria	May result in breakdown in house training, especially overnight or if left for longer periods.
Polyphagia	May increase scavenging, begging and possessive aggression over food.
Polydipsia	May increase possessiveness over water or unwillingness to stray away from water sources. Resultant polyuria may affect house training as above.
Pain, soreness or heightened sensitivity	May increase defensive behaviour and irritability, and so aggression. The dog may be reluctant to be handled or may initially seek affection then suddenly change to threat.
Lethargy or weakness	May lead to reduced motivation for interaction or exercise, or increased irritability and so aggression.

pain can vary according to its trigger and a variety of pain regulators, such as endogenous opiates, medication, mechanoreceptor activity (rubbing), emotions and stress.

Behavioural changes arising due to pain may include withdrawal, reluctance to move or perform normal behaviours, soliciting care such as through vocalization or attention seeking, withdrawal or defensive aggression if the dog is being handled or irritable. If other clinical signs are not yet apparent the role of pain in aggression may not be initially recognized.

Pain triggers activity in many areas of the brain. These include the primary and secondary somatosensory cortices in the cerebral cortex, which are the prime centres for associative learning. It also affects the limbic system, which is the emotional centre in the brain, and in particular the amygdala, which is responsible for fear and anxiety. Which centre has greatest short- and long-term influence over the dog's behaviour will depend on the pain's intensity, how readily it can be avoided, past learning and temperament. As such, its impact on behaviour can be variable and unpredictable.

Disease of the endocrine system

The specific behavioural effects of common diseases of the endocrine system are summarized in Table 7. Also see Table 6 for behavioural effects of generic clinical signs.

Disease of the nervous system

The specific behavioural effects of common diseases of the nervous system are summarized in Table 8. Also see Table 6 for behavioural effects of generic clinical signs.

Hepatic encephalopathy

Hepatic encephalopathy occurs due to an accumulation of ammonia in the blood stream caused by failure of the liver to remove it. It affects brain function, leading to listlessness, aggression, anxiety and compulsive behaviour.

Anal gland infection

Anal gland infection is reputed to mimic the pheromone produced by a bitch in oestrus. This can interfere with communicatory signals, trigger inappropriate sexual attention or underpin conflict with other dogs.

Dietary sensitivity

Dietary sensitivity refers to an abnormal response to a normal dietary component. This may arise due to an allergic (i.e. involving the immune system) or non-allergic response. Common behavioural signs of dietary intolerance are summarized in Box 2.4.

Table 7. Behavioural influence of common pathologies of the endocrine system (Overall, 2003; Mills et al., 2012).

Illness	Endocrine change	Typical behavioural signs
Hypothyroidism	Reduced thyroid function	Behavioural signs include lethargy, anxiety and increased irritability leading to increased likelihood of aggression. Behavioural effects may be seen without other physiological changes. Suggested to contribute to 1.7% of cases of aggression (Beaver, 1983).
Hyperthyroidism	Increased thyroid function	Behavioural signs include hyperactivity and increased irritability and so likelihood of aggression. Less common than hypothyroid in dogs.
Hypoadrenocorticism (Addison's disease)	Reduced gluco-corticoid +/− reduced mineralo-corticoid production	Interrupts normal stress-coping mechanisms leading to potential over-reaction to innocuous stimuli.
Hyperadrenocorticism (HAC or Cushing's disease)	Increased ACTH and cortisol production	Signs linked to chronic stress. Dysregulation of aggression and anxiety thresholds.
Testicular and ovarian tumours	Increased/decreased hormone production	Changes in the behaviours driven by the affected hormone.

Table 8. Behavioural influence of common pathologies of the nervous system (Overall, 2003; Mills *et al.*, 2012).

Illness	Typical behaviour effect
Seizures	Increased fear or likelihood of aggression. Typically post-ictal or during (potentially undiagnosed) petit mal seizures.
Brain disorders including neoplasia, encephalitis, infection, hydrocephalus or lesions	The effect will vary with the area of the brain affected. May include: • Circling or pacing • Frustration or abnormal arousal (reward centres) • Learning (reward centres) • Uninhibited rapidly escalating aggression (temporal lobe, limbic system and hypothalamus) • Interruption of sensory signals affecting normal interpretation or response to stimuli • Interruption of motor behaviours affecting normal responses • Ritualistic behaviour (lesions in the frontal lobe, internal capsule and basal nuclei, especially the caudate nucleus)

Box 2.4. Behavioural signs of dietary intolerance.

- Erratic eating patterns
- Excessive plant eating
- Coprophagia
- Pica
- Excessive yawning or stretching due to abdominal discomfort
- Excessive resource guarding due to increased value of food
- Irritability, increased anxiety or aggression, compulsions or erratic behaviour linked to changes in diet.

When considering fluctuating behavioural signs, thought needs to be given to feeding of treats and table scraps, scavenging or use of economy diets that may change in composition between batches.

Treatment often involves changing to a hypoallergenic diet that either uses low-allergy proteins, such as soy, or hydrolyses the proteins to a low molecular weight so they are no longer recognized by the body. This prevents allergic or sensitivity reactions being triggered. Wheat or lactose sensitivity may require a gluten- or lactose-free diet.

Medications

Many medications may have intentional or unintentional effects on behaviour. Any drug containing hormones or specifically intended to modify hormone function can be expected to have associated side effects. The behavioural effects of psychotropic medication are discussed in Chapter 7. The potential side effects of common medications not specifically intended to modify hormone function or behaviour are summarized in Table 9.

Nurture

The experiences of the animal from conception, through early development, maturation and decline have a significant impact on on-going behaviour.

Maternal influences

Maternal states during gestation

Development of the embryo is inextricably linked with the state of the dam. Healthy physiological development is dependent on her nutritional and health status. Any deficiencies risk leading to abnormalities or weaknesses in the neonate. Some medications or diagnostic investigations such as X-rays may increase the risk of genetic mutation during development, may interfere with development or cause pre-natal organ toxicity. Elevated maternal stress levels will also impact on development of the HPA axis and may impair normal coping abilities in the offspring. This can have a permanent adverse effect on learning, play and social behaviour.

Maternal influences post-parturition

A puppy's relationship and interactions with his dam will have an on-going effect on adult behaviour. Relevant influences are summarized in Table 10.

Table 9. Potential behavioural side effects of common veterinary medications (Notari and Mills, 2011; Mills *et al.*, 2012).

Drug	Physiological effect	Behavioural effect
Antibiotics	Elimination of bacteria	May affect bacterial content of anal sac secretions, leading to inappropriate sexual approaches by or conflict with other dogs.
Corticosteroids	Mimic or augment endogenous corticosteroids	Human and rat studies suggest intensification of stress responses during treatment with exogenous steroids leading to increased anxiety, depression, impairment of learning and memory, and aggression. Studies into the effects of steroids on dog behaviour are in the early stages and the true causality of behaviour changes seen is yet to be established. However, it is advised that the potential effects be borne in mind.
Chlorphenamine maleate	Antihistamine	May cause drowsiness, blurred vision, confusion, excitation and irritability. Acts as a serotonin and norepinephrine reuptake inhibitor so may reduce anxiety and compulsions. May disinhibit aggression.
Acepromazine	Dopamine and adrenergic antagonist for premedication, tranquilization and sedation	Reduces arousal and reward. Induces lethargy and slows reactions. Blunts decision making. May result in defensive or inappropriate aggression. Shown to cause chronic stress when used long term. Said to increase noise sensitivity.
Phenyl-propanolamine	Catecholamine mimic for urethral sphincter incompetence in the bitch post-neuter	May increase restlessness, irritability and aggression.
Ephedrine	An alpha and beta adrenergic receptor agonist for urethral sphincter incompetence in the bitch post-neuter	Stimulation of the central nervous system may lead to sleeplessness, excitation, anxiety and muscle tremors.

Table 10. Maternal influences on adult behaviour of offspring.

Influence	Discussion
Observational learning	Offspring learn from observing the behaviour patterns of their dam.
Development of stress responses	Coping behaviour of offspring is detrimentally affected by elevated stress levels and poor coping behaviours in the dam.
Conditioning	Offspring will learn from the parent through both operant and classical conditioning (see below). For example, they will learn to associate maternal pheromones with safety. They will also learn not to repeat behaviours the mother corrects.
Attachment	The quality of maternal attachments may affect exploration and confidence, and future attachments to owners or conspecifics.
Reflexes	Frustration of normal reflexes may lead to abnormalities in later life. For example, puppies that are not permitted to suckle normally may develop adult oral fixations.

Developmental periods

As puppies develop they pass through a series of periods of heightened sensitivity to certain experiences. Their experiences during each of these phases has an enormous influence on their adult behaviour. Any compromise to normal development during these phases can never be fully compensated for through training in later life. Management of early experiences is therefore critical for normal behavioural development.

Neonatal period

The neonatal period extends from birth until the puppy opens his eyes. During this period puppies are blind and almost deaf. There is little electrical activity in the brain, they have poor motor control and their responses to stimuli are slowed due to lack of nerve myelination. They are also unable to regulate their own body temperature or eliminate without stimulation.

However, they do have the senses of taste and touch at birth and so are already identifying familiar tastes and touch sensations in their environment. They can also differentiate smells, although some suggest this is through taste rather than true olfaction. Puppies are therefore thought to locate the dam by using scent/taste and their ability to differentiate between warm and cold, and soft and hard using their facial nerves. They also use their sense of taste to identify lactose in the dam's milk.

Transitional period (14–21 days)

From 2 to 3 weeks of age there is a substantial increase in brain alpha-waves and the more advanced brain structures such as the hippocampus start to develop. The puppies' sleep patterns start to show light and deep cycles and they have a fully functioning pain response. By the end of the transitional period they will have started to control their own body temperature and elimination. They will be able to stand and their eyes and ear canals will open, enabling them to see and hear. If the puppy does not experience sights, sounds, smells and tactile sensations by the end of this period the sensory system supporting neural networks will atrophy and die and their ability to do so will be permanently lost.

Socialization and habituation period (3–12 weeks)

By 3–4 weeks of age puppies have spatial perception and increasing physical control of movement such as being able to correct their balance, wag their tail and vocalize. By 5 weeks the electrical activity in the brain, nerve myelination and physical brain appearance are almost the same as an adults. Their vision, hearing and sense of smell continue to develop until they reach adult acuity at about 6 weeks. The dam will also start to wean the puppies during this period as teeth start to erupt. As the puppies' mobility, sensory ability and cognitive processes develop they start to interact with each other and to explore outside of the nest. This is their critical period of socialization and habituation.

Puppies start to recognize different species and develop affiliations to them during this period. The peak of sensitivity to making these affiliations starts as they become fully mobile at about 4 weeks and ends as they enter a period of heightened sensitivity to fear at 8–9 nine weeks. They form their filial (parental) and fraternal (sibling) attachments to the species most like themselves. This later provides the foundation for their sexual attachment. The presence of other species will not prevent normal filial identification, but if they do not meet other dogs at all during this phase they may develop a filial attachment to a substitute species, which may result in rejection of their own species when they meet them at a later time. They also form bonds with any other species they meet during this period. They have a particularly strong genetic drive to form affiliations with people and will prioritize human interaction over interactions with other puppies from a young age.

As puppies are able to discriminate between individuals of markedly different appearances, such as different genders, size, skin/hair colour and ways of behaving, they need to meet many different types of people to recognize them as all belonging to that species. This also applies to different breeds of dog, both in appearance and behavioural patterns such as play. Puppies spend a lot of time developing their social skills during this period through play. Play closely mimics agonistic and hunting behaviours. This is how puppies learn social communication and how any predatory behaviours their breed uses are switched on. They learn how to control the strength of their bite (bite inhibition) and how to share through the responses of other puppies during play. They learn submissive postures from mock fights, competition with other puppies and discipline from the dam.

Puppies also learn about their environment during this period, referred to as habituation. Exploration requires a balance between curiosity and caution to enable safe learning. As the puppies' senses awaken their curiosity is naturally triggered. However, uncontrolled curiosity puts the puppies at risk. This is therefore balanced by fear as nature's way of protecting them from excessive danger. Fear does not start to develop until about 5 weeks of age and puppies do not typically show a full fear response until 8–9 weeks, reflecting development and maturation of the limbic structures controlling fear and memory formation. Therefore any non-threatening environmental stimuli the puppies experience prior to full development of the fear response will generally be accepted as safe. However, abnormal development can interfere with this and there is evidence to suggest the onset of the fear period varies with breeds. For example it is thought to be as early as 5 weeks in the German shepherd dog.

Once the full fear response is in place the puppy will start to show some caution around new things, reducing the amount of time he is in contact with them so the likelihood he will habituate to them. The amount of time he needs to spend around the stimulus to habituate to it also gradually increases, until the heightened sensitivity to accepting new things closes at about 14 weeks.

Providing the puppy has developed normally, new stimuli experienced after this time will not necessarily be feared but will be approached with a natural caution and will be assessed and responded to according to the level of threat it poses. However, any interference with normal development may affect the puppy's long-term reaction to anything new. A lack of exposure to normal everyday triggers during the habituation period may lead to a heightened fear response in later life. Excessive stress or prevention of opportunities to withdraw from triggers may sensitize the puppy to novelty or threat or interfere with their perception they can cope with them. A chronic lack of stimulation may also lead to hyperexcitation leading to poor concentration and learning. It is suggested this may be due to the lack of normal development of the mesencephalic reticular formation, the part of the brain that controls inhibition of excitation. Alternatively, some puppies may have adjusted to a lower level of stimulation so that a subsequent normal level of stimulation has the same effect in them as a high level of stimulation would have in a normal puppy. A complete lack of even mild stressors may also be detrimental due failure of the stress response to develop at all, again risking excessive responses when the puppy is older. Ensuring the puppy is exposed to normal everyday experiences in a way he can cope with during this period is therefore critical to normal development.

Post-socialization period (14 weeks to puberty)

Development of motor and social skills continue to be honed until social maturity at 18–36 months.

At puberty the puppy will be influenced by further hormone surges, dependent on gender, which will increase sexual dimorphism. For example, the female's vulva and nipples will develop and become more prominent. The male will be more likely to show agonistic behaviour in the presence of other males and will develop increased body mass. Both genders may have peaks and troughs of hormone levels during the pubescent period, which may affect behaviour and mood until these settle and regulate. Changes in behaviour may include testing of boundaries or challenging their owners or other dogs in the house. This normally passes as long as it is neither encouraged nor met with punishment.

It is thought dogs also undergo a second period of heightened sensitivity to fear between 9 and 18 months of age, typically around puberty. This may result in a loss of confidence or sudden fear of things previously habituated to in some dogs. Most normally pass through this phase as they mature, as long as it is not aggravated or reinforced in some way. However, there is a risk that inappropriate human responses may aggravate it or that the fear itself may reinforce the behaviour, due to the distress it inherently causes confirming in the dog's mind there really is something to be worried about.

Maturity

Changes in behaviour are commonly reported as the dog reaches full maturity between 18 and 36 months. This may result in a further period of heightened anxiety as the dog no longer feels able to rely on other adults for protection or starts to challenge for things of value.

Old age and degeneration

The physiological influences and controls over behaviour undergo further change as a dog ages. Such changes may cause deterioration in learning and memory with many potential associated effects such as the breakdown of learnt behaviours (e.g. house training), failure to recognize people or places and confusion. Failing sensory function may also affect responses to the environment and generalized debilitation or reduced energy levels may affect motivation.

Age-related behaviour changes may be seen any time after the animal reaches 8 years of age, regardless of breed. They may be intermittent or mild at first but typically become more intense or frequent as the condition progresses. A more acute onset may be triggered by an event, e.g. kennelling.

Signs of brain ageing

The typical behavioural signs of central nervous system deterioration in ageing dogs are summarized in Table 11.

Causes of brain ageing

The principal anatomical changes underpinning age-related behaviour changes are reduced brain mass, thickening of the meninges and vascular degeneration resulting in reduced cerebral perfusion and so function. Death of small clusters of brain cells may also lead to disruption in normal neuronal processes. Plaques of amyloidal proteins in the brain can further cause disease either chemically or due to physical interference with cell structure.

Free radicals

Free radicals (FRs) are solitary electrons that arise as a by-product of oxidation. They can cause cell damage by attacking protein nucleic acid, damaging neuronal cell membranes and triggering DNA mutation. Removal of free radicals is reduced in old age and ageing cells are more susceptible to the effects of free radical damage. They can therefore contribute to cognitive decline.

Increased monoamine oxidase production

Monoamine oxidase (MAO) refers to a group of enzymes that break down (oxidise) monoamines, a specific group of neurotransmitters. MAO-B breaks down dopamine and the neurotransmitter phenethylamine, which is responsible for release of dopamine. MAO-B production increases in old age, so circulating dopamine levels fall, resulting in reduced feelings of reward, cognition, memory and learning.

Learning

Learning is the process whereby an animal develops knowledge from experience, which can then be used to dictate future behavioural responses. The ability of a species to learn varies. Behaviour that is controlled by learning carries risks associated with making mistakes whilst learning takes place. It is therefore in some ways inferior to unvarying inherited behaviour patterns. However, learning enables behavioural plasticity, i.e. adaptability to many situations, which makes it superior to innate behaviours in complex species.

Non-associative learning

Non-associative learning describes learning that occurs without making associations between two or more stimuli. The principal forms of non-associative learning are habituation, sensitization and perceptual learning. Habituation is the process by which an animal's emotional or behavioural response to a

Table 11. Behavioural signs of brain ageing.

Behavioural change	Discussion
Sleep patterns	Damage to the sleep centres in the brain can lead to changes in the sleep/wake cycle. This may include sleeping more in the day, agitation at bedtime and vocalization, restlessness or wandering aimlessly at night.
Loss of house-training	The effect of memory loss can lead to a breakdown of house-training. This may be seen as out of character soiling in the house, asking to go out then not eliminating or forgetting appropriate or specific places to eliminate.
Confusion	Damage to memory centres and connections in the brain can lead to signs of disorientation such as seeming lost, fear of new things, failure to recognize familiar people/places, forgetfulness, anxiety, incoordination or difficulty with normal movement, difficulty learning new tasks, slowed reactions or general confusion. In advanced cases aging dogs may perform behaviours that are out of context, e.g. growling at the wall.
Changes in social interaction	Confusion or fear may lead to irritability, heightened aggression or changes in relationships with other dogs. Reduced motivation may lead to a reduced willingness to socially interact.
Stereotypies	Anxiety or confusion may lead to development of repetitive behaviours to alleviate stress. This may include repetitive pacing or other motor patterns, repetitive vocalization or persistent licking or chewing of fur.

harmless stimulus lessens as he becomes familiar to it. For example a dog may initially sniff a new item of garden furniture but over time start to ignore it. Sensitization is where the dog's response to a stimulus becomes more intense after repeated exposure to it. For example, an animal that was previously indifferent to thunder may become sensitized to it after being shut out in a particularly intense thunderstorm, even if it did not cause him any actual harm. Perceptual learning is where a dog learns to recognize and discriminate between different stimuli.

Associative learning

Associative learning describes learning that occurs by making associations between a stimulus and an involuntary or voluntary response. Classical conditioning occurs when a new stimulus becomes paired with a stimulus that naturally triggers an involuntary physiological response. With repetition the new stimulus can trigger the involuntary response on its own. Operant conditioning occurs when an animal learns to repeat behaviour that gets a good outcome and avoid repeating behaviour that gets a bad outcome. These are discussed in more detail in Chapter 7.

Complex learning

Complex learning describes the ways in which dogs learn to recognize and categorize what things are, their relationship to other things and to incorporate new information into existing knowledge.

This enables them to learn the most appropriate response to stimuli. For example, if a dog is socialized to rabbits during his sensitive period then he will form a memory of what makes a rabbit a rabbit, primarily based on smell. He will then recognize and respond in a sociable way to future rabbits he meets, but not necessarily to other small furry animals. Complex learning may also involve making deductions about information available and using this to modify responses. Box 2.5 gives an example of behaviour that suggests complex learning in dogs.

Cultural learning

Cultural learning describes learning that occurs through interactions with others. This may include passing of information, such as by scent, or through observation and copying of others behaviour. The example in Box 2.5 also illustrates observational learning.

Motor learning

Motor learning is learning physical skills through repetition.

The Current Environment

As discussed, an animal's physiology and development will have a significant influence over its behaviour. However, it is ultimately the current environment that triggers the behavioural responses. Relevant environmental factors are as follows.

Box 2.5. An example of complex learning in the domestic dog.

When a person performs a task such as turning on a light switch their first choice is to do so with their hands. However, humans also learn a great deal by observing the behaviour of others. Researchers looking at child behaviour have shown that if a 14-month-old child sees an adult turning on a light switch using their forehead observational learning will override their genetic preference and they will copy what they see the adult do. However, they also saw that if the child watched the adult turn on a light switch using their forehead when they had their hands full, they would go back to their usual preference of using their hands. They suggested this showed the child was interpreting the available information and making the deduction that the person had used their forehead

because their hands were full. They therefore decided there was no reason to copy this if their own hands were empty.

Range *et al.* (2007) decided to replicate this experiment with dogs to see if they would also interpret the reasons for another's behaviour before deciding whether to copy it. When dogs perform tasks they will usually use their mouth. They therefore trained a border collie to pull a lever with her paw in return for a food treat. They then let other dogs observe. Those dogs that watched her pull the lever with her paw also used their paw when mimicking the task. However, those that watched her pull the lever with her paw whilst holding a ball in her mouth chose to use their mouth.

Environmental triggers

Behaviour occurs in response to current triggers. Hiding in the cupboard under the stairs not only requires the genetic temperament for or learnt fear of thunder but also the presence of thunder itself. Although this may seem obvious, the environmental triggers for behaviour can be complex and subtle. For example, a trigger may only cause a behavioural response if it reaches a certain intensity, or if it occurs in combination with other triggers. Whether a dog will respond to a trigger may also depend on other factors such as his emotional or other states at the time. Triggers can be elusive, misleading or hard to pinpoint. They may be hard for humans to identify due to differences in sensory perception. However, all stimuli are potential triggers for behaviour and all behaviour is in some way in response to environmental stimuli. These therefore always need to be considered and explored when trying to identify the reason for the dog's behaviour.

Behaviour of others

A dog's behaviour is always at least partially in response to the behaviour of those around him. For example, social behaviour requires responses from others to be successful and threat behaviour may often be in response to real or perceived threat from another, whatever the species. Therefore, when interpreting the behaviour of the dog the behaviour of those surrounding him must be taken into account.

The potential for miscommunication between dogs and people is of particular importance. Dogs and people have co-evolved to be able to interpret each other's signals and so a great deal of communication occurs successfully. However, this has limitations as humans can be poor at reading low-level canine signals and dogs still instinctively interpret most human behaviour by the laws of dog–dog communication. As such, human behaviour such as leaning over or placing a hand on the back of a dog's neck may be seen as a threat in a dog that is poorly socialized to human handling habits or that has been mistreated in the past. At the same time the human doing so may fail to recognize and respond to the dog's initial signal that he feels uncomfortable with it. This can lead to escalation of threat.

Dogs are also highly intuitive to the emotional state of others. If a dog is communicating fear this may trigger fearful or possibly defensive behaviour in other dogs around him. If humans are stressed, fearful or angry this may be perceived as a sign there is something to be worried about or may be misinterpreted as a threat. Friction between people or directed at other dogs is also a common source of stress or aggressive behaviour in dogs as they take steps to control or prevent this.

Behaviour restriction

If a dog is prevented from performing his preferred response he may be forced to take alternative action. For example, a fearful animal that is cornered is more likely to escalate an aggressive response than one that has a clear escape route.

Co-influence

Ultimately the dog's behaviour will occur as a result of all of these potential triggers and influences. They must therefore all be considered when thinking about why the dogs behaves the way he does.

3 Domestication of the Dog

Mankind has domesticated over 40 different species, all of which, by their very definition, have evolved to suit man's needs and to live under his control. In most cases these changes have made the species easier to breed, handle and care for. They may have also made them more productive or aesthetically pleasing. However, in the domestic dog (*Canis lupus familiaris*) the changes have been taken a step further. Not only have they evolved to be easier to manage, breed and set to work for us, but they have also developed an ability to interact and communicate with us in a way unprecedented in any other species. In 1863 Galton, whose research underpins the study of domestication, suggested 'The animal which above all others is a companion to man is the dog.' He goes on to say 'As the man understands the thoughts of the dog, so the dog understands the thoughts of the man, by attending to his natural voice, his countenance, and his actions.' That quote is as relevant today as it has ever been. To understand why the dog has this special role and what motivates canine behaviour we first need to understand how the dog evolved.

How Evolution Occurs

For a species to be regarded as domesticated it must have undergone sufficient change in its physiology, morphology (outward appearance) or behaviour to be distinct from its progenitor (ancestor). The process of domestication may occur in one of two ways.

In natural selection the process of domestication starts when living in closer proximity to or interdependently with man improves the progenitor species' chance of survival and breeding. This is part of the normal process of evolution and usually occurs in response to changes in the environment or in man's behaviour in ways that affect the local wild species. As the new species emerges it may be safer to have around. Man may then start to take

greater control of the species and further interbreed those that are most suited to his needs. These then become more common.

In artificial selection the changes leading to domestication are wholly controlled by man. This generally occurs where a species is already sufficiently docile or manageable for man to take control of it, either in its wild form or after a period of natural selection that has favoured traits suited to domesticity such as tameness. Over time man will then favour those individuals that better suit his needs, such as those that are larger or more fertile, causing further changes that eventually make the wild and domesticated species distinct from each other.

In both cases man's investment in caring for and rearing the new species must be to his advantage to make it worthwhile. The changes must also be 'adaptive' for the wild species, i.e. must enable continued survival and procreation, albeit in captivity.

Possible Progenitors

The domestic dog shares a genus, karyotype (arrangement of chromosomes) and mitochondrial DNA with the grey wolf (*Canis lupus lupus*), the red wolf (*Canis lupus rufus*), the Ethiopian wolf (*Canis simensis*), the jackal (*Canis aureus*, *Canis mesomelas* and *Canis adustus*) and the coyote (*Canis latrans*). It is therefore interfertile with and so potentially related to all of them.

The current consensus is that the principal progenitor of the domestic dog was the 'old world' grey wolf. However, there is continuing debate and on-going research regarding the timing and location of the first domestication of dogs and the possibility of other or combined progenitors. The detail of this research is beyond the scope of this book. However, its relevance in understanding how dog behaviour has been influenced by its ancestor and the pressures that led to its domestication are important to bear in mind.

Domestication Process

The process by which the domestic dog evolved is the subject of debate. However, an understanding of how it may have happened offers insight into the nature of the dog and how the human–canine bond became established.

Wolf cub theory

Early theories of dog domestication were based on the suggestion that humans would sometimes adopt orphaned wolf cubs. The tamest of these would then stay close to human camps as they matured and form breeding colonies, leading to a population of increasingly tame wolves. Man would then favour those that showed the most useful behaviour traits, gradually creating the variety of breeds we know today. This theory suited the historical view that man has 'dominion over' and controls all animals. However, more recent evidence suggests that even the most docile and well socialized first generation wolves remain unpredictable around humans so it is unlikely that man would have tolerated them. The chance that sufficient orphaned wolf cubs with a naturally tame tendency were adopted at the same time to enable a breeding population to form is also considered remote.

Natural selection theory

Evidence for close interaction between man and wolves and for changes in wolf morphology are seen as early as 100,000 BP, as the last glacial period got underway. The earliest evidence of the existence of the domestic dog as a distinct species is seen as the same glacial period was coming to an end, between 10 and 14,000 BP. This implies that the gradual transition from wolf to dog occurred over an extended period in which a large part of the world was covered in ice.

This has provided the basis for a theory suggesting that the shortage of resources and land space brought about by the glacial period favoured those wolves willing to live in closer proximity to man and scavenge on human waste. These slightly tamer wolves would then have formed a separate breeding population, leading to more frequent occurrence of the genes for tameness and any linked genes that came with them. As the ice age ended and mankind moved from a hunter-gatherer to a farming lifestyle, the link between man and the emerging dog then became stronger and safer, at which point man would have taken over control of their breeding and favoured those with specific traits they found useful.

Research with silver foxes (*Vulpes vulpes*) has supported the theory that tameness can be intensified by interbreeding slightly tamer foxes, resulting in foxes that are not only completely tame but also seek out human attention and affection within surprisingly few generations. The study also found that tameness was genetically linked to many physical changes such as coat colour and tail shape (Trut, 1999).

Co-evolution theory

Over the period in which the dog was emerging mankind also underwent many cultural and behavioural changes. Some of these were helped by or relied upon his close relationship with the emerging dog. Modern *Homo sapiens* are also said to show social behaviour that is much closer to that of the dog than to other primates. This is given as evidence to suggest that canine and human evolution was interlinked and that neither would have evolved as they are without the other.

Evolved Changes

Traditional explanations for dog behaviour relied heavily on the behaviour of the wolf. It is true that there are many similarities between wolf and dog behaviour, as there are between many species within a genus. However, the domestication process has also led to many changes.

Interactions with humans

Wolves socialized to humans during their sensitive period can be partially tamed. However, this remains unreliable in maturity and untamed adult wolves are timid and avoid man. Dogs also socialize to humans during their sensitive period. However, the bond formed is much more reliable and their subsequent interactions with humans go far beyond the simple process of socialization to another species.

For example, adult dogs demonstrate increased observation of and desire to follow their owner in comparison with other humans (Mongillo *et al.*, 2010) and puppies as young as 16 weeks form preferential bonds with their owners, whereas hand-reared wolves do not (Topal *et al.*, 2005). Dogs also 'catch' human yawns, a behaviour said to suggest empathy, especially from their owners (Romero *et al.*, 2013).

Dogs have also evolved the ability to read and respond to human emotions and signals. They are able to learn to read human facial expressions (Deputte and Doll, 2011) and show the left gaze bias associated with reading emotion when looking at humans but not at other dogs (Guo *et al.*, 2009). They have an ability to follow human pointing to locate food and a tendency to look to humans for help when unable to perform a task not seen in hand-reared wolves (Miklósi *et al.*, 2003). They will also copy owners' actions to obtain food or a toy even if it is contrary to the way they have learnt or been taught to do so (Kubinyi *et al.*, 2003; Range *et al.*, 2011).

These behaviours demonstrate that dogs not only socialize to humans in the way wolves do but have genetically evolved to form an attachment to specific people and to work cooperatively and under direction from humans.

Reduced dispersal

On maturity some wolf pack members naturally disperse to form new or join other nearby packs. Adult dogs show reduced desire to disperse on maturity. They will become more willing to move temporarily further away from their social group as they reach puberty, often resulting in a sudden breakdown in recall or a tendency to roam. They will also travel to find a mate. However, they do not voluntarily permanently disperse.

Hunting and diet

Wolves hunt medium to large prey in packs. Some breeds of dog still show full hunting behaviour and will hunt cooperatively. However, most dogs feed by scavenging or by seeking care from people even if stray or living ferally. The predatory behaviour of many breeds has also been changed to show only those parts of the canine hunting behaviour pattern suited to their particular role with humans (see below).

The predatory nature of wolves reflects the fact they are almost exclusively carnivorous. However, dogs have adapted both behaviourally and physiologically to the omnivorous diet that comes with scavenging and care solicitation from humans. Dogs have the genetic code for digesting starch, which is missing in the wolf (Axelsson *et al.*, 2013). Their palate has also changed. For example, they have developed a preference for cooked over raw food (Houpt and Smith, 1981), possibly as a result of cooked food constituting a substantial proportion of scavenged or begged food.

Fecundity

Dogs produce more offspring than wolves. Wolves reach sexual maturity in their second or third year, have one oestrus cycle per year and a litter of from three to six cubs. Most dogs reach puberty between 7 and 12 months, have two oestrus cycles a year and litters of between 3 and 12 pups. This change is most likely to have occurred due to artificial selection in which man favoured individuals that produced more puppies.

Communication

Wolves and dogs share many aspects of their complex visual, behavioural, auditory and olfactory communication patterns. However, canine communication has modified since domestication. Wolves generally stop barking as they reach maturity but dogs continue to do so and use a range of complex vocalizations not seen in wolves. The ability of humans to interpret them (Pongracz *et al.*, 2006) suggests this may have occurred through selection in favour of those that humans were better able to understand. Changes in appearance may also interfere with communication in some dog breeds (see below).

Breed variation

Although the early transition from wolf to dog is now widely accepted as having occurred naturally, later changes will have been strongly influenced by artificial selection by man. Initially this is likely to have occurred unconsciously, with people of the time being more tolerant of or providing better care for those individuals demonstrating traits they found useful or attractive. Over time those traits will then have proliferated and become intensified, creating the first informal 'breeds' of dog. By Roman times the diversity currently seen in dogs was already apparent and over the subsequent 2000 years dog breeds became more established and formalized. Breeds can now be loosely categorized by the original function they were intended to fulfil.

Stock movement/herding breeds

Dogs used to herd or move livestock can be drovers, musterers or tending dogs. Drovers such as the corgi herd from behind with the farmer, nipping at the heels of stock. Musterers such as border collies gather and push flocks from behind towards the farmer in front of the flock. Tending breeds such as the German or Belgian shepherd dogs work as living fences, running back and forth beside a long narrow group of livestock to keep them walking behind the farmer. They also run around grazing stock to keep them from straying. These behaviours reflect selected parts of the canine hunting sequence, combined with selection for close association with and attention to man.

Breeds used in hunting

Some breeds retain the full hunting pattern. Sight hounds are bred for speed and to visually locate, chase and kill game. Some terriers are required to locate, capture and kill prey in burrows.

Others will assist with the hunt using selected parts of the hunting sequence. Scent hounds are bred to locate prey by tracking or trailing using their heightened scenting ability, but not to chase, catch or kill it. Pointing breeds such as pointers and setters are bred to stop and 'point' at the prey with their muzzle without flushing, capturing or killing. The point may be lost if the dog gets into a habit of chasing. Flushing dogs, such as cocker spaniels for birds and the dachshund for badgers and other burrow dwellers, are bred to locate game and chase it from a hiding place for the human hunter to kill. Retrieving breeds such as golden retrievers, labradors and water dogs such as poodles are bred for watchfulness and visual acuity to see where shot game falls, a soft mouth to prevent damage and a biddable nature to return and relinquish it. Bay dogs such as the Grand Bleu de Gascogne or Rhodesian ridgeback locate, chase then hold the prey at bay until the hunter arrives to kill it. Some terriers also hold the quarry at bay underground until dug out by the hunter.

Guarding breeds

Guarding breeds have been selected to be large, intimidating and to have heightened territorial or social protective behaviour. Livestock guarding dogs are socialized to the stock they are to guard during their sensitive period, so protecting them becomes natural. Examples include the Anatolian shepherd dog or Tibetan mastiff. Other breeds, such as the chow chow and doberman pinscher, are used to protect territory or their human social groups.

Draught breeds

Draught breeds are selected to pull carts, sledges or wagons, potentially over long distances and for prolonged periods. Some are bred for speed and others for strength. For example, the Siberian husky is faster but does not have the strength or endurance of the Alaskan malamute.

Fighting and baiting breeds

Fighting and baiting breeds are bred for strength and tenacity and so persistence despite injuries when fighting other dogs or baiting other species. Examples include the Staffordshire bull terrier or shar pei for dog fighting and the bulldog for bull baiting.

Rescue breeds

Rescue breeds have been bred to find and then bring back or signal the location of lost or injured people. Examples include the St Bernard for mountain rescue and Newfoundland for people in water.

Lap dogs

Lap dogs have been bred to be small, docile and sedentary. They have an increased affiliation with and show heightened care-seeking behaviour towards people. However, it must be remembered not all small dogs are lap dogs.

Variations within breeds

The physical and behavioural characteristics associated with recognized breeds are most predictable within purebred dogs, although are also seen in crossbreeds or mixed breed dogs carrying specific genes in common with a recognized breed. The predictability of these characteristics in purebred dogs is generally good but not absolute. For example, there can be regional variations due to intensification of particular traits within local populations. In their homeland, German shepherd dogs are primarily bred for temperament whereas in the UK they are more commonly bred for appearance, leading to variations in both looks and behaviour depending on the country in which the breed line originates. There are also commonly differences between 'show' and 'working' lines of some breeds due to the different priorities of their respective breeders, resulting in distinct appearance and behaviour (see Figs 1 and 2).

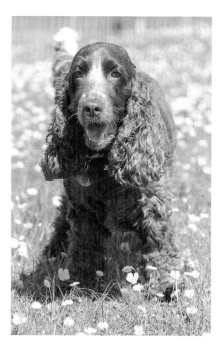

Fig. 1. Brodie: an example of a show-line English cocker spaniel.

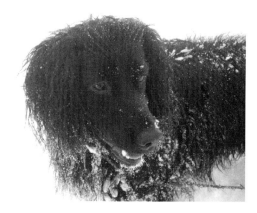

Fig. 2. Otus: an example of a working line English cocker spaniel.

Typically show lines are more fearful, and less playful and curious, making them better behaved in the show ring and less prone to aggression. Working dogs are more playful and aggressive. Natural genetic variation will further add to lack of complete predictability in breed characteristics. For example, some border collies will not even stalk or chase sheep, whereas others may complete the hunting ritual and attack or even kill them

Adaptivity of breed traits

Whether intended or not, artificial selection can give rise to traits that are not necessarily adaptive. It is common for breed traits to leave dogs wholly dependent on man, although it can be argued that this is adaptive within their current niche. Artificial selection can also result in the persistence of behaviour outside of normal ranges. This is especially likely as dogs assume an increasingly purely pet role rather than being required to fulfil a working role in which deviation would not be tolerated. Equally, the move to the pet role can make strong working drive intolerable, and some changes may benefit man but not favour interactions with other dogs, such as those that prevent a dog being able to communicate properly.

Conclusion

There is still debate about the process of dog domestication, and research is on-going. However, what is clear is that the dog has evolved to fulfil an entirely new niche living close to and dependently on man. Reference to the behaviour of likely ancestors such as the wolf to explain dog behaviour is therefore redundant. To do so is akin to using studies of chimpanzee or bonobo behaviour to understand the behaviour of humans. There is now a wealth of research into the natural behaviour of the dog whether feral, living in groups and or its natural domestic setting. Modern professional dog trainers and behaviourists now rely on this to understand, explain and modify dog behaviour rather than outdated beliefs about wolf behaviour.

4

Social, Feeding, Territorial and Reproductive Behaviour of the Dog

Social Behaviour

Social behaviour in the dog

The domestic dog is a socially gregarious species. This adaption to group living is maintained through complex social communication and cooperation. Dogs perform many group activities and the behaviour of others will strongly influence the individual. Group behaviours include social play, mutual grooming and synchronized periods of activity and rest. Territorial alarms, warnings or even aggression also typically involve all the members of the group, even if only triggered by one individual. Care-giving behaviour usually occurs from old to young, with care solicited through high-pitched vocalizations, submissive posturing and nuzzling or licking the muzzle. The latter reflects juvenile behaviour seen in wolf cubs and other immature canines intended to stimulate regurgitation of food by care givers.

Resolution of conflict

In any social species there will be times when there is conflict between two or more individuals. This is most likely to arise due to competition over possession of valued items or in defence.

During periods of conflict the primary adaptive aim of most dogs is to avoid true aggression, i.e. to avoid causing each other harm. This tendency will have been, and continues to be, favoured by evolution. Causing injury increases the risk of also receiving injury. Therefore in natural selection those individuals able to resolve conflict without being injured are more likely to survive and pass their genes into the next generation. Artificial selection also usually favours dogs that communicate without biting, as people are generally intolerant of aggressive dogs. Dogs therefore avoid true aggression through a series of communicatory signals indicating each individual's intention to escalate or back off from a disagreement, until

one backs down. The signals used are discussed further in Chapter 5.

Social structures and hierarchies

Traditionally dogs were believed to live in strict linear dominance hierarchies in which the people the dog lived with had a place. This theory suggested that all interactions between dogs (or dogs and people) resulted from the establishment of a 'pecking order' within the pack. The most senior pack member would be the 'dominant' or 'top' dog, also known as the 'alpha' or 'pack leader'. The remaining pack members would then fall in behind, each taking their place in order of seniority. Dominance was absolute and gave the 'top' dog the right to all privileges such as eating first, choosing where to sleep, passing through doorways first, leading the 'pack' when out on walks and having control over all resources such as toys or attention. Dominance also gave the 'top' dog of each gender group sole breeding rights within the group or pack.

Pack structure was said to be maintained by lower ranking dogs showing deference to higher ranking dogs. This included not trying to take any of the above privileges and appeasing if the higher ranking dog showed threat or attempted to control them. However, the dog that controls such resources has the right to breed. Therefore, given that all animals are driven by the desire to pass on their genes into the next generation, the theory also suggested that most or all dogs would try to take resources or assert control if they saw the opportunity in order to elevate their place in the pack and so the chance to reproduce. The pack leader would therefore need to continually assert his position, using aggression if necessary, to maintain his status and so the right to breed. The pack was therefore suggested to be in a constant state of tension.

This theory evolved from studies of captive wolves performed by Rudolf Schenkel in the 1930–1940s.

These studies showed a great deal of tension between successive mixed groups of red and grey wolves living in a small compound at a zoo in Germany. The stronger wolves were seen to frequently use aggression to control access to all resources and social interactions between other wolves. Weaker wolves avoided being the target of such aggression by actively deferring to the stronger wolf using appeasing (submissive) postures. Where they did not, a fight would follow, occasionally resulting in the death of the 'lower ranking' wolf.

Schenkel interpreted these observations as evidence that wolves lived in strict linear hierarchies as discussed above. He suggested the higher ranking wolves were controlling lower ranking members to maintain the right to breed, and lower ranking members accepted this by deferring. However, he described all mature wolves as having 'an ever ready expansion power, a tendency to widen, not necessarily his personal territory, but rather, his own social behaviour freedoms, and to repress his kumpans of the same sex' (Schenkel, 1946, p. 11). In short he saw all the wolves as waiting for their chance to elevate their own position and repress those of others to advance their status and so right to breed.

At that time ethologists believed that dogs had been domesticated by being tamed by man and were otherwise largely unchanged from their ancestor. They therefore concluded that Schenkel's theory of the linear hierarchy must also apply to dogs.

This led to the development of a method of canine management that relied on humans both preventing and correcting all problem behaviour by asserting their position as 'alpha' or 'pack leader'. In principle this involved controlling all their dog's behaviour and access to anything of value, and using threat if the dog behaved in a way seen to be trying to challenge for these privileges. The precise way in which this principle was applied varied between advocates. However, there are a number of common themes, which can be loosely delineated into non-confrontational and confrontational methods, as summarized in Tables 12 and 13.

More recent research has challenged the application of Schenkel's theory. However, before considering its critics it is important to understand the true definition of dominance and dominance hierarchies.

What is dominance?

Dominance is a term used to describe relationships of control and power between individuals throughout the animal kingdom. The nature of that relationship and how it is established varies according to the species, the situation and the author.

In higher mammals the term is used to describe the victor in a conflict between two individuals. For example, if there are two dogs and one bone, the dog that successfully takes control of the bone is dominant. Some suggest that each encounter leads

Table 12. Non-confrontational methods historically suggested for asserting owner dominance (these methods are no longer advocated – see text).

Technique	Examples of advice given
Control access to food	Only feed after the owner has finished eating, eat a biscuit or pretend to eat from the dog's bowl before feeding, keep a hand in the dog's bowl as he eats or routinely take food away, by force if needed.
Control access through doorways	Prevent dogs walking ahead through doorways, using commands or force depending on the source. 'Walk through' dogs lying in doorways.
Prevent pulling	Prevent dogs walking ahead of humans when on lead, or off lead without the explicit permission of the 'pack leader'.
Control access to resting places	Prevent dogs sitting or sleeping with owners and access to higher resting places such as sofas, chairs and beds. Some also advise sitting in the dog's bed to 'claim' it.
Control height	Dogs are not allowed upstairs or to stand in a higher position than their owners.
Control interactions and behaviour	Dogs should not be allowed to initiate interactions. Any attempt to do so should be ignored. Some advocate the dog should be ignored at all times other than when training or that all the dog's behaviour should be controlled and access to anything the dog values prevented other than when given explicit permission by the 'pack leader'.

Table 13. Confrontational methods historically suggested for asserting owner dominance (these methods are no longer advocated – see text).

Technique	Description
Use of dominance or threat postures	Maintaining eye contact with the dog until he averts his eyes or rolls on to his back. This may include standing over the dog in an intimidating stance or growling at the dog.
Scruffing, muzzle grabbing and alpha rolls	Grabbing the dog by the scruff and shaking him, grabbing him by the muzzle or forcibly rolling him on to his side/back until he stops resisting. These are said to mimic wolf corrections.
Imitation bites	Sharply jabbing the dog with a hand shaped like a claw or with two or three fingers. Some also suggest prong or pinch collars imitate a bite.
Physical punishment	Suggestions include hitting with the hand or an object, overtly kicking, applying the heel to the underbelly of the dog or biting (especially the ear).

to one party being dominant and the other submissive and so a dominance/subordinate relationship can occur from the first time two dogs have a dispute. Others believe dominance is only earned after one dog has repeatedly won against the other resulting in an established relationship. In this case the loser typically starts to defer to the winner without the need for him to use threat.

In this type of conflict it is important to recognize that the winner is determined by a huge number of factors including physical strength, emotional state, past experience and how much each individual wants the resource being disputed. It can also change over time and vary between resources, situations and from day to day. As such, whilst in every conflict there will always be a winner and a loser and a pattern may be established in some cases to avoid conflict, it does not follow that the same dog will always win or will win in every situation. Dominance therefore is not necessarily absolute and is not a personality trait. It also does not suggest that the desire to win is anything other than the desire for that object and the dog's belief he can win it. There is nothing in this to suggest doing so is part of a desire for 'alpha status' or an attempt to control all resources to maintain status or breeding rights.

What are dominance hierarchies?

Where dominance relationships become stable they can be said to have formed a hierarchy. The precise relationships between individuals in a hierarchy can vary. One example is the linear hierarchy in which each individual is placed in rank order with animal A senior to all others, animal B

subordinate to animal A but senior to all others and so on. A triangular or circular hierarchy is where seniority over one individual does not necessarily lead to seniority over all those in the group. For example, member A may be senior to member B, and member B may be senior to member C. However, member C may be senior to member A. A despotic hierarchy is where a single 'alpha' controls the behaviour of all others, who are equally subordinate (see Fig. 3).

As who wins in a conflict can change, dominance hierarchies may also vary in their stability and rigidity. Relationships may become established and remain unchanged over time (stable) or may constantly change (unstable). Equally one individual may always win (rigid) or the winner may vary between situations (fluid). This further demonstrates that dominance and any resulting hierarchies are not absolute and are not due to personality traits.

Application of dominance and hierarchies to the domestic dog

The traditional dominance hierarchy-based theory of wolf and dog behaviour suggests dogs live in a rigid but unstable linear hierarchy, in which dominance over a subordinate is absolute and a tendency to higher ranking is a personality trait.

Although this theory arose from studies of captive wolves it is now recognized that non-captive wolves form packs as family groups and do not control each other's behaviour or all resources to maintain breeding rights. More importantly it is also recognized that dogs are now sufficiently distinct from wolves that using wolf behaviour to explain dog behaviour

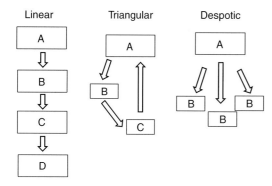

Fig. 3. Types of hierarchy.

is unreliable. Therefore the only acceptable way to evaluate whether the dominance hierarchy theory described above applies to dogs is to look at recent research into dog behaviour.

A recent study of feral dogs failed to show formation of any kind of stable hierarchy. They formed loose packs that shared territories, often based on kin groups, and challenges were made between males during breeding seasons and by females when protecting pups. However, beyond this few dominance/submission rituals were observed and there was no clear order of control or deference. Studies of communities of neutered domestic dogs also failed to show any kind of structured hierarchy (Bradshaw *et al.*, 2009).

As such there is no evidence to suggest that domestic dogs attempt to form hierarchies or to control resources and the social behaviour of others in order to maintain alpha status or breeding rights.

What are the alternatives?

An alternative model of canine social and conflict behaviour suggests that the likelihood there will be a dispute, and who will win, is primarily based on a combination of the value of the resource to each individual and their perceived ability to win in a competition.

The value of the resource will depend on how important it is to the individual's survival and how freely available it is. It will also be affected by the individual's perception of the resource. For example, a dog that is fed dry food every day may be prepared to escalate a conflict for a fresh bone but will not for his daily ration, whereas a dog that is underfed may be prepared to challenge even for the dry food. Alternatively, a dog that is well nourished

and has free access to a bowl of dry food every day but has little other stimulation may be prepared to challenge over a toy as a prey substitute or attention from the owner.

The likelihood a dog feels he can win if he chooses to challenge will depend on his physiological state, past learning and all the other factors discussed in Chapter 2. For example, a dog that has previously lost to a particular dog may be less likely to escalate aggression against the same or similar dogs in the future, whereas if he previously won he will be more confident of doing so.

Once two dogs have had a number of similar encounters they will often establish a pattern of low-level threat and deference to avoid further pointless disputes. However, this is subject to change and does not automatically apply to relationships with other dogs or different situations with the same dog. It therefore does not imply a hierarchy or established 'alpha' position.

This alternative theory accepts that dogs do have disputes over things of value to them, that the one that wins is said to be dominant and with repetition that may become an established relationship. However, it also recognizes that relationship can vary according to the resource, may change over time and where there is a group the relationships of winners and losers over different resources do not form a strict linear pattern.

More importantly it reflects that conflicts are about specific situations or resources. They are not about controlling resources or others' behaviour to maintain status or breeding rights.

Why does the traditional theory prevail?

Even in the 1980s researchers were starting to recognize that rank reduction methods did not work (Knol, 1987). However, it is still very common for people to use the dominance hierarchy model to explain and modify dog behaviour, even among some professionals. It is therefore very likely clients will have heard of or used this method and may believe it works. Given all the evidence against it, why is this the case?

One of the attractions of the method is it is very simple. It offers clients a set of clear rules that are easy to follow and require no specialist knowledge or discretion to apply. It may also 'appear' to work in some cases. Application of dominance rules may be the first time there have been any boundaries put in place for the dog's behaviour and relationship with his owner. This may bring some unruly behaviour under control or provide predictability that helps the dog better understand what he is expected to do. However, although this does appear to support the theory, these changes occur due to learning the consequences of behaviour rather than assertion of status. As such, given there are other simpler and clearer ways to get the same effect and the risks associated with rank reduction methods (see below), the alternatives are preferable.

Apparent efficacy can also sometimes be achieved through the use of the more confrontational methods often advocated (see Table 13). In some cases this may occur as a result of the dog learning that his behaviour leads to being emotionally or physically punished and so avoiding repetition. More commonly it occurs due to general fear of the owner causing the dog to avoid interaction or any non-essential behaviour, or due to 'learned helplessness'.

Do dominance methods do any harm?

It could be argued that if rank reduction may appear to work in some cases then it is worth trying. However, it can do a great deal of harm in many cases, some of which may be irreversible.

Many of the more confrontational methods associated with rank reduction (Table 13) involve causing the dog pain or making the dog fearful through intimidation or the threat of pain. This contravenes three of the RSPCA and ASPCA's five freedoms. It also runs the risk of triggering defensive aggression (Herron *et al.*, 2009). As the methods do not reflect known dog behaviour patterns they cause confusion. This makes human behaviour unpredictable to the dog, making him less able to judge it and so more likely to react defensively to it, both at the time of the corrections and in any future interaction with people. This puts the owner, trainer and anyone associated with the dog at risk (also see Chapters 6 and 7).

Many dominance-based theories recommend distancing the dog and owner relationship, e.g. ignoring or not showing affection to the dog. This may not only affect fulfilment of the dog's natural need for social interaction potentially leading to anxiety or depression, but may also interfere with fulfilment of the owner's needs as discussed in Chapter 1. In extreme cases this may lead to rehoming or euthanasia.

Even where the most innocuous methods are used (see Table 12), if the method fails to address problem behaviour this may prolong the compromise to the dog and/or owner's welfare as the problem persists. In some cases it may also lead to rehoming or euthanasia of the dog if the owner feels the problem is intractable or loses patience.

Therefore, as there are so many other ways to correct problem behaviour there is no point in taking the risks associated with rank reduction methods. Alternative methods are discussed in more detail in Chapter 7.

Feeding Behaviour

Dogs are referred to variously as omnivores or facultative (i.e. optional) carnivores, depending on the source. They still have the dentition of a carnivore and do not require dietary carbohydrate to survive. However, their digestive system has evolved to digest grains (Axelsson *et al.*, 2013) and their typical diet will normally consist of a mixture of animal- and plant-based foods.

In the western world food acquisition in most dogs occurs through a combination of opportunist scavenging and care solicitation. Most pet dogs are provided with food by their owners and dogs have developed very effective strategies for encouraging this, such as pestering at routine feeding times and begging when humans are preparing or eating food. It is also natural for them to steal unguarded food and most need to be actively trained not to do so. Their opportunist nature means many dogs' eating habits are not controlled by drives of satiation and hunger and so they will take food whenever the opportunity arises, although this can be affected by the overall availability of food and the breed.

Most breeds of dog still show parts of the canine hunting behaviour pattern, as outlined in Table 14. However, this tends to be redirected on to inanimate objects or is shown in a form that means they do not actually hunt, kill and consume prey. For example, the pug typically does not show the desire to hunt, having instead evolved to seek care and so food from its owner. The border collie still shows some stages of hunting behaviour such as 'eye', 'stalk' and 'chase' but no longer tries to locate or (all being well) grab, kill or dissect. In the absence of sheep this will often be directed on to balls or other moving objects. The ragging and dissection of toys also reflects the kill and dissection bites of the hunt, and dogs that enjoy retrieving or carrying things are showing the 'grab' part of the hunting pattern without the kill and dissect.

Table 14. The complete canine hunting pattern.

Hunting stage	Description
Locate	Location of prey is usually by sight or scent, although may also by audition.
Orient or give 'eye'	Once prey is located the canid will freeze and observe in silence whilst deciding when/which individual to target.
Stalk	A silent and slow approach intended to get closer to without alerting the prey.
Chase	Once the prey is aware, stalking will escalate to a chase.
Grab	If the canid cannot immediately give a kill bite he may initially grab and hold the prey until he or a pack member can do so.
Kill	Canine species and dog breeds vary how they kill. This may be a bite to the ventral neck to puncture blood vessels or evisceration. Others may shake small prey violently (rag) or bite the dorsal neck to fracture the spine.
Dissect	Once the prey is dead it will then be dismembered and eaten. This may include tugging with fellow pack members to break it up.

Territorial Behaviour

Domestic dogs are a territorial species. Their core territory consists of their den, typically their home and garden. Their home range extends to any place regularly visited. This may include exercise areas, such a local park or field, a workplace or another home regardless of to whom it belongs. Dogs that are given sleeping places separate to their owners, such as in a kitchen or outhouse, may occasionally see this area as a separate core territory and may defend it from their owner.

Dogs identify their social group members and any regular visitors known not to pose a threat and will greet them on arrival. If any other individual tries to enter the territory this may trigger an alarm or defensive reaction. This usually starts with barking to alert and solicit support from other members of the social group and to make the invader aware of their presence and willingness to defend the territory. It may then escalate to higher levels of threat to make the invader go away, depending on circumstances and the individual.

The intensity with which the dog will defend its territory will vary with breed and temperament. Some breeds have been artificially selected to show increased territoriality. Dogs that have been poorly socialized, have anxiety disorders, are fearful of strangers, have been encouraged by owners (sometimes inadvertently) or who have other behavioural problems may also show increased territorial behaviour.

Reproductive Behaviour

A common outcome of the domestication process is increased promiscuity and fecundity (reproductive potential). The domestic dog reaches sexual maturity, has more frequent breeding seasons, produces larger litters and is much more promiscuous than its ancestor. Most dogs' mating behaviour is driven solely by hormones with minimal mating rituals, mate selection or social controls and no prolonged associations or pairings. Some dogs may show sexual dysfunction but this is usually due to poor socialization, inhibition by the presence of another dog challenging for the right to mate or some other behavioural interference.

5 Canine Senses and Communication

Communication is the process of sending and receiving information to and from another individual. This information is then used by the receiver, alongside all the other influences discussed in Chapter 2, to drive or change their behaviour. Signals are sent through vocalization, body language, pheromones and action signals in dogs, and are received via the special senses. We will therefore consider communication and the special senses together.

Species Variation in Communication

All creatures have their own specialized forms of communication. They each evolve the physical aptitude and genetic drive to sense and communicate with the world in the way that best suits their niche. In simple species giving and understanding communicatory signals is largely driven by genetics. In more complex creatures communication is also honed during socialization and learning. For example, the canine 'play bow' (see Fig. 4) is a genetically coded innate behaviour in the dog. However, it will not become an established part of the puppy or older dog's behaviour unless he is exposed to other puppies or dogs to learn the social rules for using it.

Dogs have evolved to live as man's companion. This has resulted in an improved ability to read each other's signals. For example, dogs can follow human pointing from 4 months of age and are able to read human expressions. Their vocalizations have also become more complex to communicate with humans, and people seem to have a natural ability to understand these. However, there are still huge gaps between dog and human modes and methods of communication, and differences in the purpose of signals we have in common. Problems with communication are therefore perhaps one of the biggest causes for conflict between the two species. The more we can learn how dogs communicate the better chance we have of resolving these conflicts.

Smell

The dog's principal method of communication is smell. Dogs use scent to identify individuals (human and canine), determine gender and even recognize another's mood. Canine olfactory ability massively outstrips that of the human. They have up to 30 times greater olfactory epithelial surface area, linked by up to 60 times as many sensory cells to a 40 times larger olfactory bulb than that of humans. Many breeds are also able to simply inhale much larger quantities of air than people can. Canine behaviour patterns are designed to maximize scent collection and analysis as described in Table 15, although both physiological and behavioural scent collection ability varies with breed.

The scent of a specific item is made up of many different individual scents. For example, a favourite toy may smell of the rubber it is made from, its owner's sweat, the dog's own saliva, the grass it was sitting in overnight and the slug that passed over it in the night. Some of these smells may change, but enough stay the same for it to be identified not only as a rubber toy but also the specific rubber toy the dog left out the night before. The dog's reliance on smell for identification of and attachment to humans makes our scent particularly important to them.

Pheromones

Dogs use pheromones as part of communication. Pheromones are endogenous chemicals that carry messages. They vary between species and are normally only perceptible to others of the same species. Once absorbed they have a specific innate behavioural response according to their purpose. This response occurs independent of learning.

Pheromones are detected by the vomeronasal organ (VNO). This is a paired organ in the hard palate behind the incisors, which opens into the incisive canal and connects the mouth cavity and the nasal fossae. The VNO may be activated by odours, such as the presence

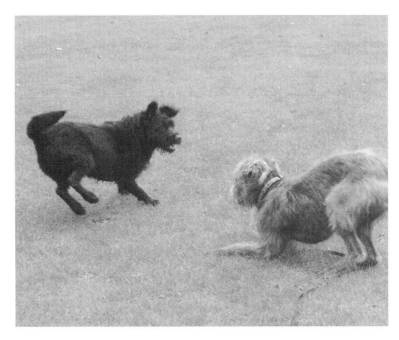

Fig. 4. The canine play bow (photograph courtesy of Laura Wyllie Dog Training).

Table 15. Scenting behaviours in the domestic dog.

Behaviour	Description
Scent location	Dogs initially locate scents using rapid head movements and sniffs. Exhalation force can throw up dust and particles to release scent chemicals.
Scent following	Dogs follow scent using slower head movements and slower deeper sniffs. They determine direction by the intensity of the odour. On the ground they zig-zag to keep within the 'corridor' of strongest scent concentration. In the air, where scent is more quickly spread, they follow scent upwind. If they lose the scent they 'quarter' the ground until they pick up the trail again. They may use a combination of scents to track movement, e.g. the scent of the person alongside the scent of broken vegetation.
Scent matching	Dogs can link a smell located in the environment to the individual leaving the mark if met later, even at a different location.

of urine, or by scenting behaviour in others. Activation triggers a behavioural response intended to increase absorption. In the dog this may be seen as tonguing: lifting the head and repeatedly pushing the tongue to the roof of the mouth whilst salivating and chattering the teeth. Dogs are also seen to taste the air by moving the head from side to side whilst drawing back the lip commissures. Once within the VNO the pheromones are absorbed and transported by pheromone-binding proteins from glands surrounding the VNO to receptors in the VNO body. Impulses are then transmitted to the limbic system where they alter the dog's emotional state. Table 16 summarizes the parts of the body that produce pheromones and their key activities.

Sound

The dog's ears open at around 19 days and start to reliably respond to sound at around 25 days of age.

Dogs hear a frequency range (pitch) of between 20 Hz to at least 45,000 Hz. They hear best at between 200 and 15,000 Hz. For comparison, humans can hear between 13,000 and 20,000 Hz and hear best between 1000 and 4000 Hz. Sonic devices intended to modify dog behaviour typically operate at between 20,000 and 60,000 Hz. They therefore cannot be heard by people but can be heard by dogs. Dogs with sound sensitivity may find these products aversive. They will also be affected by sonic pest-control devices, which work on similar frequencies. Dogs do not hear at greater intensity (loudness) than humans.

Dogs are better able to discriminate and localize sound than humans. This is due to the mobility of the pinna enabling them to 'catch' sounds, and greater development of the neurological systems that process information taken separately from each ear to determine direction and distance in the auditory centres of the brain.

Dogs generate vocalizations for a number of reasons. These are summarized in Table 17. Typically, higher pitched vocalizations are intended to increase social interaction, whereas lower pitched sounds carry more threat and so are intended to make the target withdraw.

Although humans can learn to interpret most canine vocalizations, they cannot match the ability of other dogs to read subtler meaning. In a recent experiment performed by Farago et al. (2010), recordings of growls were played from behind a screen as a dog approached an apparently unguarded bone. The growls ranged from a play growl, a defensive growl and a possessive growl. Although the latter two sounded very similar to the human ear the dog only backed away from the bone in response to the possessive growl. We must therefore keep in mind the limitations of human ability to interpret subtle variations.

Table 16. Region of production and activity of principal canine pheromones (Mills *et al.*, 2012; Stevenson and Kowalski, 2012).

Region of production	Action
Facial glands	Signal social behaviour
Ear	Appeasines from the ceruminous and sebaceous glands, signal safety and reassurance
Interdigital glands	Territorial marking and alarm
Inter-mammary sulcus	Appeasines thought to orient neonates and identify areas of safety
Urogenital region	Vulval, preputial and urinary tract secretions signal reproductive receptivity and territorial marking
Circum-anal glands	Transmitted via the anal glands by raising the tail or depositing on to faeces. Communicate identity, territorial marking and alarm. Bacterial composition also plays an important role in communication involving anal sac contents

Table 17. Motive for vocalization in the domestic dog.

Motive	Discussion
Communicate with social affiliates that are out of sight	Dogs bark, howl or whine to let other dogs or their human owners know of their whereabouts. This is a social behaviour intended to maintain contact with the rest of the group. It may often trigger other dogs within earshot to bark back, even if they are not part of the social group. Dogs left home alone will often bark to alert their owner to their whereabouts.
To sound the alarm	Dogs will bark or possibly growl to let other group members know of an event or intrusion into the territory.
Communicate an emotion, state or desire	Dogs will use a variety of vocalizations to communicate a range of emotions, states or desires. These include pain, fear, anxiety, frustration, play incitement or expressions of excitement or fun.
Aggression avoidance	Vocalizations such as growling or aggressive barking are often used at various stages of aggressive interactions to try to avoid the conflict reaching the point of injury. This is discussed more in Chapter 6.

Vision and Touch

Vision

Dogs rely less on their sense of vision than their hearing or sense of smell. The tapetum at the back of the eye maximizes visual acuity in low lighting by reflecting and fluorescing available light to brighten dark images. The dog's vision is therefore better than a human's in darkness. However, vision in daylight is markedly less effective than that of a human. Vision in low light is comparable between the two species (Miller and Murphy, 1995).

Dogs have a wider field of vision than humans and some binocular vision, i.e. overlap of images from both eyes to form one image. The total field of vision and area of overlap varies between breeds according to the position of the eyes in the head. Peripheral vision may range from 240 to 290° and binocular vision may be between 60 and 116°. For comparison, the human field of vision is 180° and binocular range is 140° (Miller and Murphy, 1995) (see Fig. 5).

The rod and cone combinations on the dog's retina offer less clarity than humans enjoy. A typical dog's acuity is considered to be about a quarter of that of a human in daylight, with certain breeds commonly being myopic (short sighted).

In one study, 53% of German shepherd dogs and 64% of rottweilers were myopic. Long-distance images are clearer if they are moving, but it must be kept in mind that the ability of small dogs to see at distance may be affected by obstacles that larger dogs or humans can see over (Miller and Murphy, 1995).

Dogs can see in colour but do not have the same colour range as people. It is thought that they can see the blue and yellow colour spectrums, alongside shades of grey, but cannot see red or green. These are instead likely to also appear as shades of blue or yellow, which may be indistinguishable from the true colours of this spectrum (Miller and Murphy, 1995).

Visual development is complete by 5–6 weeks. Puppies' eyes open at 2 weeks but they can initially only see light and dark. They are able to discriminate shapes from around 25 days and are thought to have fully functioning vision by 6 weeks of age.

Touch

As a social species the domestic dog's tactile system is highly developed. It is able to sense movement, pressure, vibration, temperature change and changes in balance in others. Touch as a form of communication

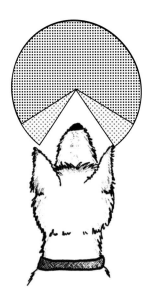

Possible canine range of peripheral vision dependent on breed

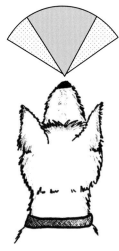

Possible canine range of binocular vision dependent on breed

Fig. 5. Ranges of peripheral and binocular vision in dogs dependent on breed.

is common in social species and is recognized as a method of both maintaining social bonds and of punishing or controlling through the threat or infliction of pain.

Visual and tactile communication

Forms of canine communication that use vision fall under the umbrella term of body language. This can include changes in body posture, proxemics and motor actions.

Postural changes

Changes in body posture can indicate emotion or intent. Movement of the pinna and tail, maintaining or avoiding eye contact, widening or narrowing of the eyes, tensing or relaxing muscles, shifting body weight, changing body position, piloerection and exposing the teeth are all used in canine communication.

Proxemics

Proxemics refers to the position the dog chooses in relation to the target for its signals. For example, the dog may approach, may withdraw or may actively avoid being close to the target even if encouraged to do so. The method of approach may also be important: stalking can be a predatory behaviour although it can also occur in play. Approaching indirectly, such as in a curve, is a passive behaviour intended to signal a friendly intention whereas a direct approach can be seen as threatening.

Action signals

Action signals refer to movements performed by the animal with a view to communicating emotion or intent. Some action signals rely on touch.

Interpretation of Communication Signals

Canine communication is subtle and complex. Humans can learn to read canine signals to understand a dog's emotional state or intention. However, it will take time to be skilled at doing so. People spend years subconsciously learning how to interpret human body language as they grow up, and yet still get it wrong. Therefore when trying to learn to read canine body language it is important to keep in mind that it has many variations and complexities

that must be learnt and taken into account when making interpretations.

Considerations when interpreting signals

Meaning of signals

Communication signals send messages to another about the signaller's emotional state or intention, or request the other to behave in a specific way. For example, a dog that lifts a paw with his tail tucked is letting the other dog know he is fearful, he intends to withdraw and would like the other dog to stay away.

However, many signals have the potential for multiple meanings. A lifted paw in a dog that is leaning towards another with a relaxed sweeping tail can be an incitement to play. Individual signals therefore cannot be read in isolation. All of the signals a dog shows must be looked at together and the interpretation made from their combined meaning.

Morphology

Dogs come in many shapes and sizes. The morphology of some breeds prevents normal signals being used and surgical interventions such as docking can interfere further. Therefore it must be borne in mind that some dogs may be trying to send a signal but it is not being seen because either they cannot do so or it is not marked enough to be noticed. For example, an English springer spaniel can only move the very base of his ears back so this signal is not as noticeable as it would be on a dog with erect ears such as a German shepherd dog.

Breed signals

The signals chosen may vary between breed. Dogs often rely on their typical breed behaviours when worried, or may play in different ways according the parts of the hunting pattern they have been bred to show. For example, border collies often stalk when they are greeting socially or can herd other dogs when they are worried by them, including nipping at their heels.

Confusing or conflicting signals

Signals used may sometimes seem to contradict each other, what the dog is doing or simply not fit the pattern. This may be because the dog is in emotional conflict and so may be sending mixed signals or keep switching between them. For example, a naturally sociable dog that has become fearful of other dogs may mix play solicitation with low level appeasing or threat to say 'I want to play but I am worried' or 'I want to play – but don't mess with me or I will stick up for myself.'

Furthermore, although we can generalize about how dogs communicate there will always be individual variation, just as there is with people. This may be due to failures in socialization, faulty learning or simple idiosyncrasies. Occasionally the behaviour may be truly abnormal, e.g. when the animal is suffering from a neurological condition or has suffered extreme deprivation during developmental periods.

Interaction between signallers

When interpreting signals it is important to remember that they are invariably partly in response to signals being received from others. Apparently inconsistent, unpredictable or inappropriate behaviour may therefore sometimes have been triggered by inaccurate interpretation of or inappropriate behaviour by others. For example, a dog may roll on his back to appease (see Figs 6 and 7). However, this is commonly misinterpreted as a request to 'tickle my tummy', the act of which can then cause the dog to growl when they feel their appease signal has not worked. On the surface this behaviour may seem unprovoked. However, recognizing how

the dog interpreted the human's approach makes it an entirely predictable response.

Social greeting and play behaviour

Social greeting and play behaviours are intended to indicate a desire to get closer to and interact with the target for the signals, be they another dog or person. Figure 8 illustrates the common signals used in this situation, although this is not exhaustive. The design of the figure is intended to show how communication involves a combination of signals and is fluid. Some signals may be seen in any social situation whereas others are specific to polite greeting, play incitement, play maintenance or termination. The combination of signals each dog uses will vary according to their own personality, the situation and the actions of the other. All interpretation must include consideration of the variations discussed above. The body language discussed is also depicted in Figs 7 and 9–20.

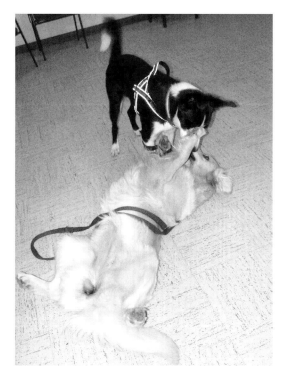

Fig. 7. A dog rolling over to play. Here the dog is relaxed, flat on her back with her legs spread. She is happily looking directly at the other dog and making contact with a paw (photograph courtesy of Laura Wyllie Dog Training).

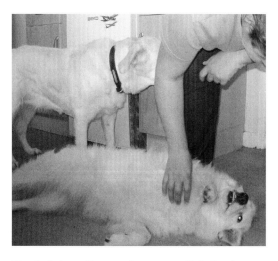

Fig. 6. A dog rolling over to appease. Note the dog has only partly rolled on to his back and has an averted gaze.

Chapter 5

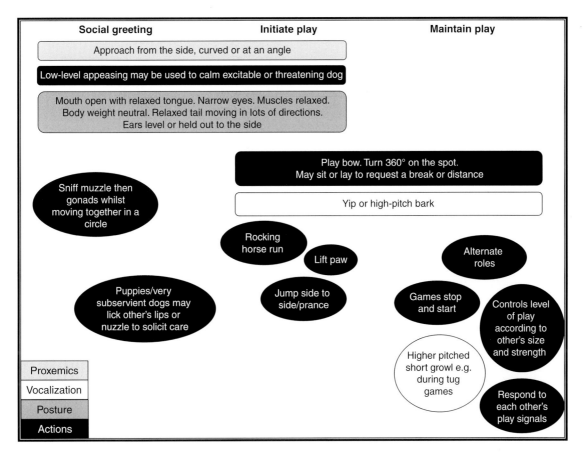

Fig. 8. Communication used in social greeting, initiation and maintenance of play.

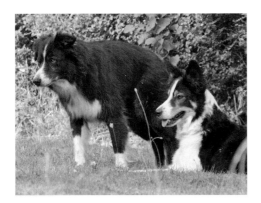

Fig. 9. Quinn and Sonny watching a puppy from a distance. Note the relaxed face and open mouth of Quinn (on the right). This suggests he is comfortable and open to friendly social interaction. However, Sonny (left) is much tenser with a hard stare, closed mouth, head tucked and body stiff and leaning forward. This suggests he is not comfortable with the approach of the puppy.

Monitoring play

Even if two dogs are both friendly free play should be supervised to ensure it is even and enjoyable for both dogs. Play is preceded by play signals such as a play bow, 'rocking horse' approach, hopping from side to side, lifting a paw or sometimes lying or stalking. Once underway games tend to follow periods of often intense activity such as romping or chasing, interspersed with brief periods when both dogs stop for a moment then restart. Both dogs have relaxed muscles and fluid body movements during this break, e.g. sweeping tails and open mouths. They may also show mild appeasing behaviours, such as narrow eyes, or more play signals. The roles in the game will alternate so both may chase or be chased, roll on their back or be on top. Bigger or older dogs should control their play to accommodate smaller or younger dogs (see Figs 18–20).

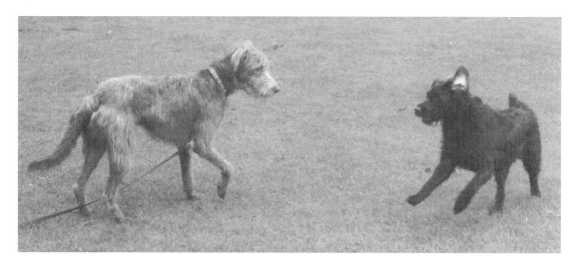

Fig. 10. Two dogs approach. Note how the approach is indirect, indicating a friendly greeting. If a dog approaches face to face or at a right angle this generally suggests threat (photograph courtesy of Laura Wyllie Dog Training).

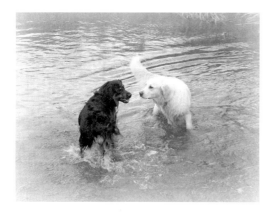

Fig. 11. Circle greeting. Here the dogs again approach indirectly and curve their bodies to show they mean no harm. Also note the relaxed faces and ears and open mouth of the dog on the left (photograph courtesy of Laura Wyllie Dog Training).

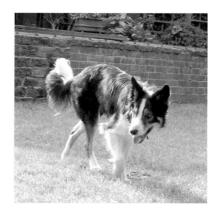

Fig. 12. Quinn approaches in play. This border collie is adopting typical breed behaviours in play. However, the open mouth, relaxed leg and sweeping tail show this is play not threat.

Watch all play signals and if you see either dog showing signs of fear, anxiety or repeatedly appeasing, the same dog always on top or chasing as the other tries to get away, excessive mounting, one dog being cornered or repeatedly pinned down or being pinned down for more than a second or two, or there are any signs of threat, interrupt the game. Excessively noisy play also suggests either fear, threat or over-arousal and so should be interrupted. If you are not sure if play is acceptable it

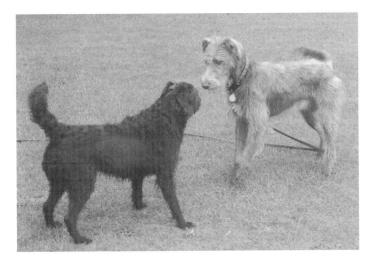

Fig. 13. A nose to nose greeting. Dogs typically sniff noses when they first greet. The spread legs of the dog on the left, paw lift of the dog on the right and the tail movement also show this is friendly (photograph courtesy of Laura Wyllie Dog Training).

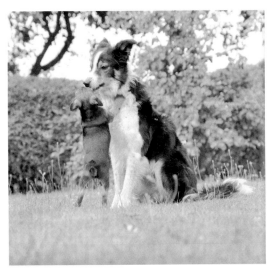

Fig. 14. Another nose to nose greeting. Slug (left) wants to greet Quinn but cannot reach him with four feet on the ground. He therefore gets on to his hind legs to do so. This is what dogs are trying to do when they are jumping up.

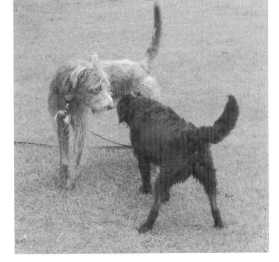

Fig. 15. Sniffing genitalia. Sniffing genitals is normal behaviour after sniffing noses. This provides the dog with additional information (photograph courtesy of Laura Wyllie Dog Training).

can help to separate the dogs and hold the more boisterous dog whilst leaving the other loose. If the quieter dog tries to restart the game it suggests he is enjoying it.

Agonistic signals

Agonistic signals surround situations of conflict or concern, typically where the dog feels he must defend himself or something of value. This may be due to (perceived) threat from the target for his signals or a learnt expectation that this situation may lead to threat or attack. All the signals are intended to try and keep the target away or ask them to withdraw in a bid to avoid true aggression, i.e. conflict that involves injury. However, if all the signals fail some dogs will ultimately escalate to biting the target in a further attempt to make them withdraw.

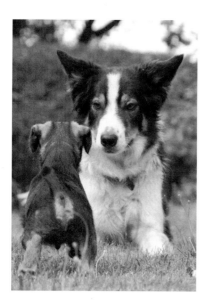

Fig. 16. Calming ears. Here Quinn uses level ears to try and calm Slug's excitement.

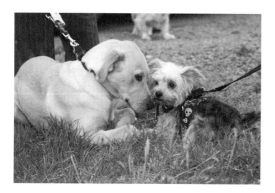

Fig. 17. Calm greeting. These dogs are showing gentle appeasing or 'calming' behaviour on greeting including laying down and avoiding direct eye contact. Their relaxed bodies and close proximity suggest they are not worried by each other (photograph courtesy of Tom Worle Photography).

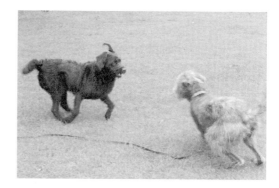

Fig. 18. Jumping side to side. These dogs are initiating play by jumping from side to side. Note the floppy ears, loose tails and bent legs (photograph courtesy of Laura Wyllie Dog Training).

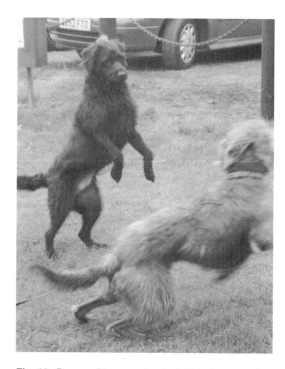

Fig. 19. Pounce. Play can also be initiated by pouncing on the spot (photograph courtesy of Laura Wyllie Dog Training).

Figure 21 illustrates the signals that may be used in this situation, although is not exhaustive. The design is intended to show how communication involves a combination of signals and is fluid. Some signals may be seen in any conflict situation whereas others are specific to appeasing or threat behaviour. Each dog will make individual choices about which signals to use dependent on their temperament, the situation, the behaviour of the other and all the factors discussed in Chapter 2. Most dogs typically start somewhere in the middle and then choose to escalate to higher appeasement or threat if lower signals do not work. If that fails they may decide to

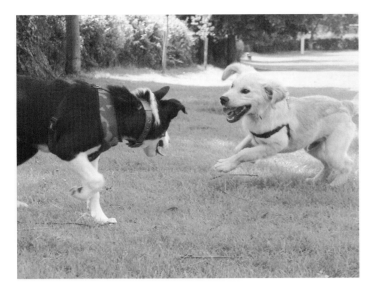

Fig. 20. Play posture. Taken mid-play, this shows the on-going relaxed face with open mouth, bent legs, and floppy ears seen when both dogs are enjoying the game (photograph courtesy of Laura Wyllie Dog Training).

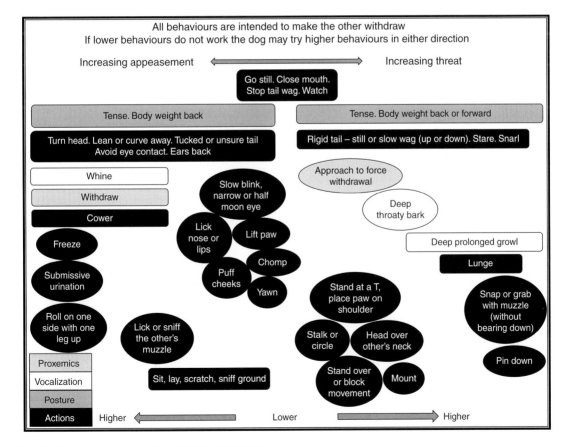

Fig. 21. Communication used in agonistic interactions.

change direction from threat to appeasing or vice versa at any point, possibly skipping straight to higher levels when doing so. If the dog has used low-level signals in the past which have failed to deter the target he may choose to skip these during later encounters and escalate straight to higher level signals, again in either direction. All interpretation must include consideration of the variations discussed above. The body language discussed is also depicted in Figs 6, 9 and 22–34.

The one thing all these signals have in common is that they indicate the dog feels under threat and that he needs to defend either himself or something of value to him. When this type of behaviour is seen in the veterinary practice it is usually due to either current staff behaviour or a learnt expectation of being handled in a way the dog sees as threatening. This is invariably unintentional. However, the dog will not understand this and so simply sees a threat he must try to defend himself against.

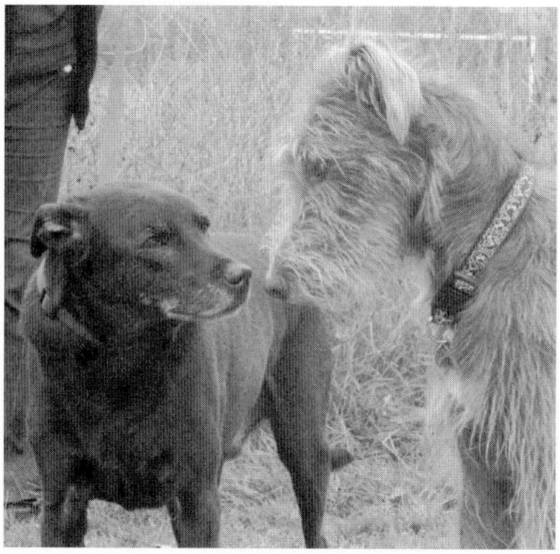

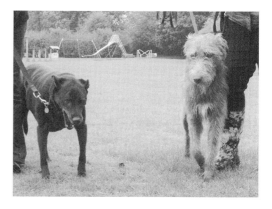

Fig. 24. Appeasing yawn. As the dog takes a step closer he also yawns as a sign of stress and appeasement (photograph courtesy of Laura Wyllie Dog Training).

Fig. 22. Appeasing greet. Rufus no longer enjoys playing with other dogs. Here he narrows his eyes, looks to one side and puts his ears back to show he is uncomfortable with this dog's attention (photograph courtesy of Laura Wyllie Dog Training).

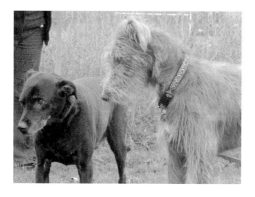

Fig. 23. Turn away. Rufus then turns away to further show he would prefer this dog to back off (photograph courtesy of Laura Wyllie Dog Training).

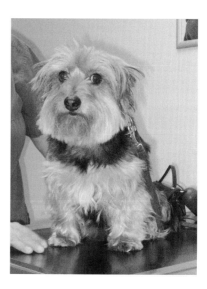

Fig. 25. Whale or half-moon eye and furrowed brow. The crescent of sclera and furrowed brow show how worried this little dog is.

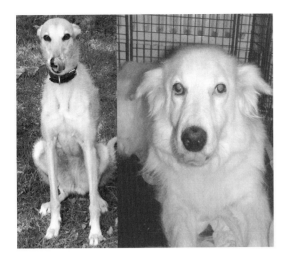

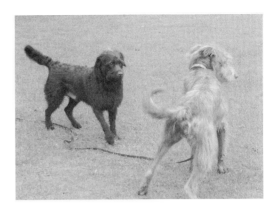

Fig. 26. Appeasing nose and lip lick. The dog on the left is appeasing by narrowing her eyes and licking her nose. The dog on the right's concern is indicated by a lick of the lips, pulled back ears and the crescent of sclera.

Fig. 27. Turn away. The brown dog on the left looks stiff as he approaches. Ralph, on the right, appeases him by turning away to avoid conflict (photograph courtesy of Laura Wyllie Dog Training).

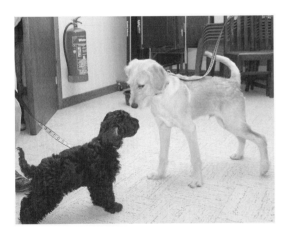

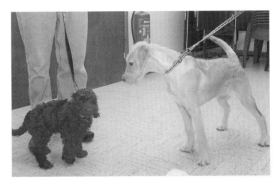

Figs 28 and 29. Another appease turn-away. The white dog on the right is stiff and standing over the black dog on the left in the first image. As he leans forward further the black dog backs off, lifts a paw and turns away to ask him to give a bit more space (photograph courtesy of Tom Worle Photography).

Figure 35 illustrates an example of how a dog may initially choose to use low-level appeasing behaviours in the practice and how this may change according the behaviour of the person handling him. It shows how if signals are recognized early, steps can be taken to dispel the dog's perception of threat and prevent escalation to aggression. It also shows how being able to avoid the dog feeling the need to show even low-level appeasing behaviour will reduce the dog's perception of the vets as a worrying place to be and so the likelihood of aggression on subsequent occasions. A dogs use of aggression and its associated communication is discussed further in Chapter 6.

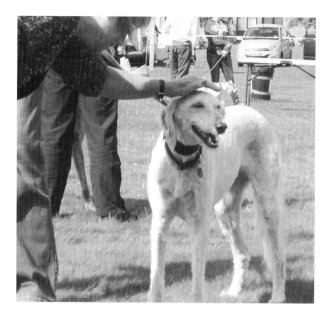

Fig. 30. Appeasing a 'threat' approach by a human. This lady has approached this dog in a straight line and is touching the back of her head. She clearly intends this in a friendly way. However, the dog is showing she finds it worrying by turning her head away, leaning away and narrowing her eyes. This is her way of asking the lady to back off.

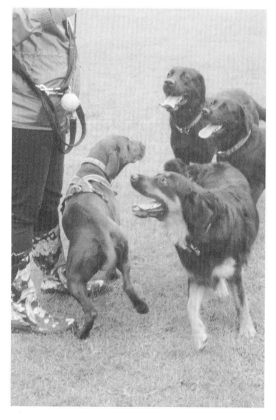
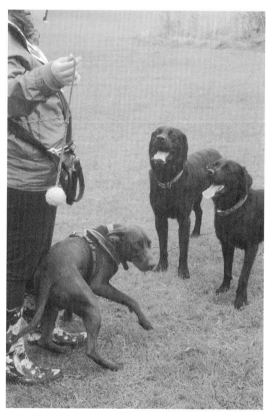

Figs 31 and 32. Strong appease. The brown dog on the left is showing strong appeasing in response to three dogs approaching at speed. They are in fact more interested in the ball. However, it shows how a dog's behaviour is a response to how they perceive a situation, not necessarily how it is intended (photograph courtesy of Laura Wyllie Dog Training).

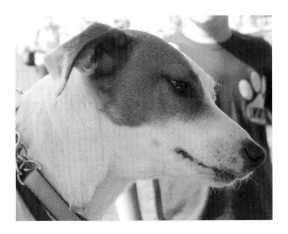

Fig. 33. Facial tension. Note the stillness and rigidity, the fact the lip commissures are pulled forward a little and head slightly tucked. Although slight, these indicate that dog is uncomfortable with the situation.

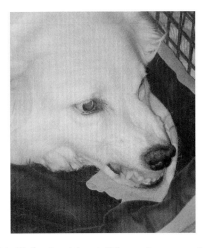

Fig. 34. Higher level threat. This can be seen not only in the drawn-back lips but also the hard stare, lowered body posture and wrinkled nose.

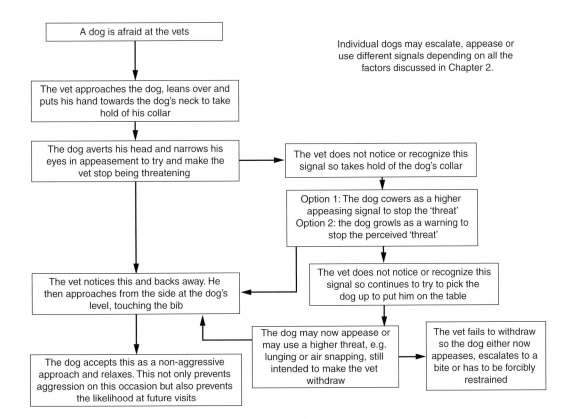

Fig. 35. Appeasement and escalation of aggression in response to the target's signals.

6 Problem Behaviour

Dogs may show problem behaviour for many reasons. In most cases, behaviour the owner sees as a problem is in fact part of the dog's normal everyday behaviour that he simply has not yet been trained not to do. This would include things like jumping up, mouthing and pulling on the lead. These are discussed more in Chapter 14. In other cases the problem behaviour may be more complex. Behaviours such as aggression, compulsions, anxiety or chronic or inappropriate fears or phobias are not necessarily abnormal. They are usually the dog's way of coping with an adverse situation, or arise due to past experience, faulty learning or problems with the dog's interpretation of the current environment. However, even though they are theoretically adaptive to the dog's current situation they are also a threat to the welfare of both the dog and the owner. Living with a dog showing these types of behaviours can be emotionally distressing, can interfere with the owner's freedom and quality of life and can be dangerous in some cases. They also indicate the dog is emotionally distressed in some way. They therefore need to be addressed.

The diagnosis of the causes for and treatment of these types of problems is complex and therefore needs to be referred to an accredited specialist. However, it will help the veterinary team better support their client if they have an understanding of common problem behaviours and why they tend to occur.

Aggression

Aggression is the most common reason for people to seek help with their dog's behaviour and is very likely to be the most common reason people relinquish or euthanize pets on behavioural grounds. Understanding and responding appropriately to canine aggression is therefore an essential skill for all members of the veterinary team not only to protect both themselves and their clients but also to protect the dog.

What is aggression?

There are many different formal definitions of aggression. There are many more personal or colloquial interpretations of what aggression is. When defining the term it must be remembered that many of the behaviours that surround it are in fact communication intended to avoid real harm. For clarity the term aggression will be used here to collectively describe all behaviour used to try and control the behaviour of others through the threat of or actual harm, and for predatory aggression. The term 'true aggression' will be used to discriminate when the dog is causing actual harm, i.e. biting. Behaviour intended to make others withdraw without the threat of harm, such as cowering, withdrawing and lip licking, will be referred to as appeasing behaviour. Behaviour that threatens harm without actually causing it, such as staring, growling or snapping, will be described as 'threat'. When discussing all these behaviours collectively they will be referred to as 'agonistic behaviour', being the term for behaviour used during conflict (see Fig. 36).

Aggression may be predatory or emotional (affective), each of which has very different drives and is governed by different parts of the brain.

Predatory aggression

Predatory behaviour is governed by activity in the lateral hypothalamus. It therefore has very little sympathetic 'fight or flight' nervous system activity. It instead stimulates similar reward sensations to eating and drinking. Predatory aggression can be differentiated from emotional agonistic behaviour as summarized in Table 18.

Predatory drives are stronger in some breeds than others. Many breeds have either completely lost their predatory drive or have had it modified to be of use to man, e.g. herding or retrieving breeds. However, those breeds that have been allowed to retain their full hunting behavioural pattern, such

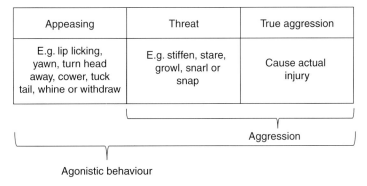

Appeasing	Threat	True aggression
E.g. lip licking, yawn, turn head away, cower, tuck tail, whine or withdraw	E.g. stiffen, stare, growl, snarl or snap	Cause actual injury

Aggression

Agonistic behaviour

Fig. 36. Definitions of terms used when describing aggression.

Table 18. Behavioural differentials for predatory aggression.

Signal	Discussion
Lack of threat or sound	The aim is to avoid alerting the 'prey'. Both approach and attack are therefore normally silent. There are no agonistic signals.
Predatory patterns	Predatory behaviour patterns are normally seen, although some steps may be missed. The attack will typically be aimed at the neck or ventral abdomen, and often involves shaking.
Unresponsive to appeasement or withdrawal	The prey will be pursued beyond a boundary. The attack will not stop despite agonistic signals.

as Jack Russell terriers and lurchers, may still have a strong desire to kill and will derive great pleasure from it. The more often the behaviour is performed the more established and pleasurable it will become. Predation in some dogs is also stronger when in groups and some breeds only tend to hunt in a pack, e.g. fox hounds.

Predation may be directed towards any species to which the dog is not socialized. The tendency to show predatory aggression and the choice of prey will vary with breed, size and genetics. The most common targets are typical prey species such as birds, rabbits and hare, rodents, squirrels or small deer. Some dogs may also show predatory behaviour towards cats. Exceptionally rarely this behaviour may be directed at babies or small children, or at other dogs. If a dog has not been socialized to babies or toddlers their strange sounds and jerky movement may mimic that of injured prey. Prospective or new parents should not be unduly alarmed with such information as incidents require a combination of a poorly socialized animal and a high prey drive. However, whilst any aggression to children is much more likely to be affective, early introductions must be monitored for any sign of predatory behaviour.

Aggression to other dogs is also much more likely to be due to defensive behaviour. However, predation on other dogs, whilst rare, does occur. The predatory drive may also underpin chasing and attacking inanimate objects, e.g. bicycles or skateboards.

Emotional (affective) aggression

Affective aggression differs from predatory aggression in that it has an emotional drive behind it. It is regulated by the medial hypothalamus, periaqueductal grey matter (PAG) and the amygdala, among other structures. The PAG is linked to sensations of anxiety, distress, panic and terror. The amygdala is linked to fear, anxiety and emotional learning. It also has strong links to the 'fight or flight' and fear responses, and the punishment centres in the brain. As such, dogs displaying affective aggression are emotionally distressed.

Use of aggression for protection or to acquire or retain a resource is a normal adaptive part of canine behaviour. However, true aggression is risky as the target may retaliate with equal force. It also is not evolutionarily adaptive for dogs to be aggressive to humans: they rely on us for survival and if they show aggression that is put in jeopardy. It is therefore normal for dogs to avoid aggression where possible through appeasement.

The most common reason for dogs to show aggression, whether to humans or other dogs, is if they feel they, their offspring or a member of their social group is under threat. This may be a genuine threat, such as an attack by another dog or genuine hostility from a human. Alternatively it may be a perceived threat when none actually exists such as where the dog has become sensitized to or fearful of a trigger. For example, if a dog develops a phobia of men wearing hats they may anticipate danger from every man wearing a hat that they meet and so show aggression to them to pre-empt the attack they are expecting.

Defensive aggression can also arise due to miscommunication between dogs or, more commonly, people and dogs. People will often behave in ways that are similar to how dogs behave when they are threatening each other. For example we tend to lean over dogs to greet them, or touch them on the back of the head or neck, both of which mimic canine threat behaviour (see Chapter 5 and Fig. 30). Most dogs learn from a young age that people tend to do this and mean them no harm. However, if a dog was not properly socialized to these ways of handling as a puppy, if they have been sensitized to this by past mishandling or if they are in a situation in which they feel fearful or in danger they may interpret such behaviour as a threat and react accordingly. Sensitization to this handling is particularly likely following use of the dominance techniques, which typically involve using this type of behaviour as a threat (see Chapter 4 and below).

Dogs may also show aggression to defend or, less commonly, acquire a resource. Resources can include food, toys or other articles the dog has come to value. They can also be territorial such as their home, preferred resting places or regular exercise areas. Dogs may also regard owners or companions as a resource that they are at risk of losing and so must protect from being taken from them.

Whether they will defend a resource primarily depends on the value of the resource to them. This is determined by a combination of what it is and how freely available it is, or has been in their past. For example if food is scarce, or a dog has been deprived of food in the past, he may be willing to fight for even a crust of bread. However, if food is plentiful this is less likely and the dog either will not compete at all or will only compete for highly prized items, such as bones or human food.

Use of aggression also depends on the dog's perception he can win, which in turn can be affected by things like his perception of his strength compared to the opponent, the threat or appeasing behaviour shown by the other, the outcome of past disagreements and his level of confidence.

Hostile aggression

It is recognized that humans may use aggression for reasons other than defence or control of resources. For example, they may do so out of anger or revenge. The only immediate benefit in doing so is the release of the negative emotions triggered by the target. However, there may be more complex adaptive social values to such behaviour, such as inhibiting people from performing behaviour likely to trigger such responses.

The human tendency towards anthropomorphism may sometimes lead people to think a dog's behaviour is driven by hostility. For example, it is common for people to feel a dog has bitten them because he dislikes them, or because he is annoyed with them for something they may have done previously. Theories of linear dominance hierarchies also imply hostile behaviour when suggesting a dog will use aggression to control another's behaviour simply to assert seniority.

Whether animals show hostile behaviour is debatable. There is currently no evidence to support the suggestion they may, although this remains to be fully explored. There is, however, extensive research to support our understanding of dogs using aggression in self-defence or to control resources of immediate value. Such explanations can invariably be seen in all instances of aggression once properly explored. Therefore, given the lack of evidence for hostile aggression, this explanation is the more reliable one.

Aggression thresholds

Defence and control of resources are the key triggers for aggression. However, there can be considerable variation in the use of aggression in response to them, both between dogs and on different occasions in the same dog. This can be affected by the value of resources, the dog's perception he can win, past experiences, the behaviour of others, current emotional state, the intensity of triggers, his perceived alternatives and all the other influences discussed in Chapter 2.

One way to illustrate how these influences come together to determine whether and what level of aggression a dog will use in a specific situation is to use the theories of 'bite thresholds' and trigger stacking.

'Bite threshold' is an established term used to describe the point at which a dog will use aggression (Donaldson, 1996). Some factors will push the dog closer to his threshold, i.e. will make it more likely he will show aggression. Others will reduce the dog's threshold for aggression, i.e. will reduce how much it takes to push the dog to that point. The combination of where the dog's threshold is and what factors exist to push him closer to or over it determines whether the dog will use aggression in a given situation. It will also influence the level of aggression used. Trigger stacking refers to numerous triggers occurring together and pushing a dog over this threshold in combination when they would not on their own.

This way of explaining aggression can be illustrated by using an example of a dog that has a fear of thunderstorms, men and sticks (see Fig. 37). In this example the dog has never shown aggression before, yet unexpectedly bites a man in the street. Figure 37a shows the dog's normal threshold for aggression. It also shows that although the dog is a little bothered by each of the triggers, none is enough to push him over his threshold on its own. He may very well be showing appeasing behaviours in these situations, but if the owner is unaware of these he may be oblivious to the fact the dog is bothered by any of the triggers. Figure 37b shows how if the dog unexpectedly gets caught out in a thunderstorm one day and a man passes by with a walking stick, the three triggers may combine to push the dog over his threshold, causing him to bite. To the owner this may seem 'out of the blue', especially where lower level fear or appeasing behaviour used in the past have not been noticed. The decision to use aggression may also be affected by things like being on a lead and so unable to escape, how close the man is and the behaviour of the owner or the man towards the dog. Figure 37c shows how influences such as pain may reduce the dog's threshold, causing him to use aggression in response to a single trigger alone.

This is a very simplistic model and the number of influential factors in the real world may be huge. Each dog's baseline for aggressive behaviour will also vary, according to all the factors discussed in

(a) A dog has a mild fear of men, thunder and sticks. Each bring the dog closer to but not over his threshold.

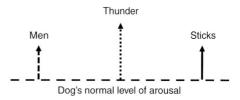

(b) The dog is on a walk in a thunderstorm and passes a man with a stick. These three triggers in combination push him over his threshold.

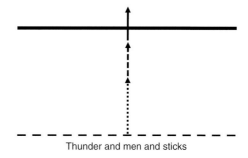

(c) The dog has hurt its leg and is in pain reducing his threshold. Thunder alone is now enough to trigger threat or true aggression.

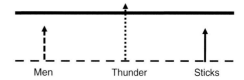

Fig. 37. Bite thresholds and trigger stacking in the domestic dog.

Chapter 2. However, it serves to illustrate how varying influences interact to cause an animal to show aggression in one situation but not in another often seemingly similar incident.

Escalation of agonistic behaviour

The type of agonistic behaviour used is partly affected by the combination of triggers, as discussed above.

However, it can also be affected by the current behaviour of the target or past experience in similar situations.

If a dog is worried by something he will typically start by using a low-level appeasing signal, such as turning his head or body away, licking his lips, narrowing his eyes or yawning (see Fig. 21). The next step will then depend on the target's response. If the target also shows appeasing behaviour this will usually signal the end of the conflict. However, if the target does not change their behaviour, or is seen as using higher threat, the dog may then show a stronger appeasing behaviour, such as cowering, walking away or even rolling on to his back. Alternatively, at any stage the dog may change tactics and try threat behaviour instead. Dogs controlling resources usually start with a low-level threat.

The threat used initially is often subtle. The dog may become still, stiff and very focused on the target. He may also use changes in body posture such as standing at right angles to the target, putting his head or paws over the target's back or neck or standing over the target if size permits this (see Fig. 21). The next step then depends on the response of the target, and the dog's willingness to use aggression as discussed above. If the other party backs off the dog may also do so. However, if they do not, or they are perceived as retaliating with higher threat, then the dog may also try using equal higher threat such as barking or growling or, if this does not work, escalate to snarling, snapping or ultimately true aggression. The dog may equally at any stage decide they are not prepared to escalate the threat further and revert to a lower level of threat or to appeasing behaviour.

Even at the higher levels of threat or true aggression, such as a dog fight, or sustained attack on a person, the dog will normally continue to read and assess the other's behaviour and decide whether to persist or back down. For example, if the dog realizes they are unable to sustain the attack or the other is stronger they may back off. It is also usual for the dog to back off if the target withdraws or appeases. Rarely neither party will appease and the fight will continue until broken up or sufficient injury has been inflicted for one of the parties to no longer be able to fight. It is also possible for one party to appease but for the other to persist with the attack, failing to respond normally to their opponent's capitulation. This is rare and abnormal.

One way of depicting how dogs may escalate from appeasing to threat and potentially true aggression is the 'ladder of aggression' (see Fig. 38). This model visually shows how dogs will start by using appeasing behaviours associated with the lower rungs and will only escalate to higher threat behaviours if these fail to work. Individuals may vary in the exact order and speed of their progression, some may escalate part of the way up and then climb back down again and some dogs may learn to skip rungs if they have failed in the past. However, the image helps illustrate the principle that they start with signals intended to avoid threat, progress to using threat to avoid true aggression and only resort to true aggression if less risky behaviours fail.

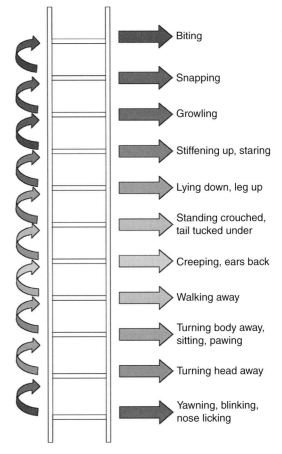

Fig. 38. Ladder of aggression (Shepherd, 2002). (Reproduced with permission from the *BSAVA Manual of Canine and Feline Behavioural Medicine*, 1st edn. © BSAVA.)

Fears and Phobias

Fear is normal and adaptive. To be successful in life animals must have a balance of confidence and curiosity. They will never learn about their world if they are not driven to explore it and they will fail to thrive physically and socially if they are not confident enough to interact and assert themselves. However, uncontrolled curiosity may be dangerous and excessive confidence may lead a dog to take undue risks or use levels of threat that put them in unnecessary danger. At normal levels, fear provides a healthy dose of caution to balance curiosity and to inhibit excessively confident behaviour.

The physiology of fears and phobias is governed by the amygdala, the part of the brain responsible for the regulation of emotions and the 'fight or flight' response via the hypothalamus (see Chapter 2). Fears are placed into context and recalled to affect future behaviour via the hippocampus and cortices.

The sensations of fear are caused by the fight or flight response, which motivate and enable the animal to withdraw from or defend itself against the threat. Their unpleasantness also serves to motivate the dog to do so in similar situations in the future. The latter primarily occurs by creating classically conditioned (unconscious) associations between the fear and the stimuli associated with the cause of it. These may be direct characteristics of the trigger, such as the size or colour of the dog or person that triggered the fear, or other simultaneous stimuli such as location, time of day or people present. Fear can also spread to things that are similar to the original trigger or associated stimuli. For example, if fear becomes conditioned to a location it may then spread to any location that shares similar characteristics. Dogs also learn to avoid fearful stimuli operantly. If they learn that certain behaviours result in something happening that makes them afraid, they may consciously learn not to repeat it. However, to what degree they do so depends on the level of fear triggered (see Chapter 7).

Although fear is normally adaptive and necessary it can cease to be functional if it interferes with the dog's normal behaviour or occurs in response to things that are not actually likely to cause harm. It is also harmful if it causes long-term stress or anxiety, both of which are detrimental to welfare.

The point at which fear becomes a phobia is the subject of debate. However, a phobia is generally accepted to be a more intense and perhaps less rational fearful response to the trigger.

One of the reasons fear can become inappropriate is because it is self-reinforcing. Fear of triggers that are genuinely harmful will naturally persist. Fear of things that are not should normally pass through habituation. However, in some cases the unpleasant sensations of the fear may not only prevent this from happening but also further reinforce the fear as the dog finds each exposure unpleasant simply due to the fear itself. For example, if a dog is attacked by another dog in the park he may then become fearful of going to that park, even though the other dog is not there and he is never attacked again. Repeated visits without any further unpleasant events should enable the dog to stop being worried. However, in some cases the unpleasant sensations of fear the dog feels whilst at the park can be enough to make him see the park as an unpleasant place to be without any further truly harmful experiences occurring. The reasons why a dog may respond abnormally fearfully are summarized in Table 19. Common triggers for fear are summarized in Table 20.

Anxiety

Anxiety is the expectation of danger or a distressing event in the absence of a specific trigger or indication it is about to happen. If it is mild and transient it is an adaptive response that motivates the animal to be cautious in potentially threatening situations. This not only enables the animal to take steps to avoid potential threat on that occasion but it also facilitates learning to improve future prediction and so avoidance. However, if it becomes a chronic state this has welfare implications.

Chronic anxiety

The key factors that lead to chronic anxiety are the same as those that lead to excessive or unjustified fear with two additions.

Chronic exposure to a fear trigger

If a dog is repeatedly exposed to a fear trigger over a period of time he may become chronically

Table 19. Common causes of susceptibility to heightened fearful responses.

Cause	Discussion
Poor socialization or habituation	Lack of proper socialization and habituation can interfere with discrimination between threatening or non-threatening stimuli, especially to new things. It can also affect the dog's ability to cope effectively with new or worrying stimuli.
Genetics	Some breeds have been selectively bred for traits that will cause them to have lower or higher fear thresholds than others. Certain individuals may have a genetic predisposition towards fearful reactions.
Maternal influences	Puppies that have been raised by fearful dams may show higher levels of fear. It is adaptive for the puppy to follow the dam's signals about what is threatening, but is unproductive if the dam's behaviour is inappropriate.
Allelomimetic behaviour	Dogs will sense if another is worried or fearful and take this as an indication there is something to be worried about. This is especially true of their owner.
Disease	Hormonal disruption, such as to the HPA axis, or disruption of neural pathways or processing may lead to inappropriate or abnormal responses or learning, which may persist even after the disease has been corrected.
Sensory impairment	This will interfere with normal interpretation of stimuli, increasing reactivity.
Impaired coping ability	This may be due to physical disability, emotional dysfunction or environmental circumstances (e.g. being confined).
Increased vulnerability	An animal's fear response is increased if they are in pain or injured or otherwise feel vulnerable.

Table 20. Common triggers for fear in the domestic dog.

Possible trigger	Description
Noises	Dogs have increased sensitivity to sound and a strong neural link between sound and the fear centres in the brain. They are therefore predisposed to sound sensitivity. They are particularly sensitive to sudden noises that they are unable to identify. Common triggers include fireworks, thunder and gunshot. Other triggers include loud vehicles (lorries, buses, tractors, etc.), household appliances (washing machines, vacuum cleaners, fridges, etc.) and people shouting. Apparently generalized anxieties can be due to noise phobia.
People	This may be generalized but is typically more specific, e.g. strangers, house visitors or people of certain ages, gender, appearance or behaviour.
Other dogs	This may be generalized but is more commonly specific, e.g. dogs of a certain size, colour, breed, behaviour or in specific locations. Dogs that have not socialized outside of their own breed (e.g. belonging to isolated breeders) may be fearful of all dogs other than their breed.
Locations or situations that predict pain	Places that are associated with fear triggers, e.g. a place where they have been attacked by another dog, have been injured or strongly punished, groomers or at the location of electric fences. Unavoidably they may also become fearful of the veterinary surgery due to association with being unwell or in pain when there in the past, the essential administration of unpleasant treatments or need to use force when handling.

anxious due the constant expectation it may recur at any time. A common example of this is when dogs are frequently physically punished, leading to the constant expectation they may be punished again. This is discussed more below and in Chapter 7.

The inability to predict or control a fearful stimulus

Being able to predict when an aversive stimulus will occur enables an animal to take evasive action such as avoidance, changes in behaviour, appeasement or self-protection. However, exposure to recurrent threat or distressing stimuli that the dog cannot identify the cause or source of makes it unpredictable. Being unable to predict when a distressing event will occur, and so being unable to take steps to avoid it, can lead to chronic anxiety. This often happens when dogs are punished incorrectly. If the dog cannot work out the reason for the punishment he cannot prevent it. This results in punishments that not only fail to change behaviour but also lead to anxiety as the dog fails to be able to predict when they will occur and so avoid them. This can in turn lead to impulsive or compulsive behaviour, aggression or learned helplessness.

Separation-related problems

Dogs may show many unwanted behaviours when left alone. Most commonly this is elimination, excessive vocalization or destructiveness. Some dogs may also show anorexia, excessive salivation, hyperactivity, self-trauma or general signs of fear. Occasionally dogs may also show compulsion or aggression towards owners as they try to leave.

Such behaviours are often automatically attributed to anxiety. However, there may be many causes for them, which must be eliminated before anxiety or distress is diagnosed. These are summarized in Table 21. Reasons why dogs may be predisposed to true anxiety on separation are summarized in Table 22.

Problem behaviour in an owner's absence can also be aggravated if the dog is punished when the owner gets home. It is common for an owner to do this in a bid to correct the behaviour or out of frustration at the mess or damage, especially if they feel the dog 'looks guilty' when they get home and so 'knows he has done wrong'. However, the delay between performance of the unwanted behaviour and the punishment means the dog will not understand why this is happening. This may then create anxiety when the owner is out due to fear of the anticipated punishment on his or her return. It can sometimes help persuade owners not to do so if they understand that the 'guilty look' is in fact a natural appeasing response to their undoubted annoyance rather than any understanding by the dog that he has done anything wrong (see Box 6.1).

Compulsive and Other Coping Behaviours

Compulsive behaviour (sometimes referred to as stereotypy) describes any behaviour that occurs repeatedly with no immediate function or purpose. The most common compulsive behaviours are motor behaviours such as pacing, tail chasing or shadow chasing. Dogs may also flank suck or repetitively lick a part of the body without a physical reason, sometimes to the point where the target tissues are traumatized. Other compulsions include hallucinations such as fly snapping or watching imaginary insects on the floor

Table 21. Potential causes for problem behaviour when left alone other than anxiety.

Sign	Possible cause
Destructiveness	May be due to play, boredom or exploration (especially in young dogs).
Vocalization	Dogs bark or howl to locate social group members and to enable others to locate them. Barking as or just after the owner leaves is common and most dogs then settle once they realize the owner is not going to take them along or return. Prolonged barking suggests greater distress or inability to cope without the owner. Barking may also be triggered by outside stimulation, e.g. doorbells, passers-by or cats outside of a window. Older dogs may start to vocalize excessively due to cognitive dysfunction.
Elimination	The dog may not yet be house trained, even when fully mature. Even if the dog asks to go out when the owner is there they may not have learnt they are required to wait until the owner gets home if they feel an urge to eliminate when alone. It may also arise due to illness or cognitive dysfunction.
Self-trauma and hypersalivation	May be caused by underlying illness.
Frustration	Many dogs are frustrated at being left behind, which is managed differently to true anxiety.
Others	Separation may aggravate other problem behaviours without being the principal cause for them. Examples include compulsive behaviours, aggression, fear of specific triggers or chronic anxiety. Occasionally the behaviour may be attention-seeking without the animal being truly anxious or distressed at the absence of the owner.

Table 22. Reasons for predisposition to anxiety at being left.

Reason	Discussion
Lack of habituation	Dogs are social animals that would naturally stay together given the opportunity. They therefore have to learn to accept not always being able to be with their owner. Most dogs learn this as puppies. If they do not, separations may be initially traumatic for them when they are older.
Impaired coping mechanisms	If the dog's ability to cope with stress is impaired, perhaps due to problems with early development or chronic stress, they may react excessively to separation.
Repeated re-homings	Dogs that have been abandoned or re-homed by a previous owner, even if for very valid reasons, may be sensitized to a repeat and so become distressed when left. This fades over time in many such dogs.
Excessive reliance on the owner	If the dog relies on the owner to cope with stress or triggers for fear he may become distressed when the owner goes either in the presence of the fear trigger or if they are expecting it. However, contrary to traditional belief, this is not triggered by spending too much time with the dog or allowing them to sleep on the owner's bed.

Box 6.1. Research showing a dogs appeasing behaviour when owners come is not due to guilt (Vollmer, 1977; Horowitz, 2009; Hecht et al., 2012)

It is common for a dog to lower his head, tuck his tail and sneak away if caught doing something his owner feels he should not, or if simply found at the scene of an earlier 'crime'. It is also common for this to be interpreted by many humans as a sign of guilt. This is due to its similarity to human expressions of guilt, such as avoiding eye contact and lowering the head, and our knowledge that people do this when they know they have done wrong and are seeking forgiveness. However, this is a misconception.

We know that dogs lower their head, avoid eye contact and withdraw to 'appease' a known threat. Research has also shown that when dogs behave this way when their owners return after absence it is triggered by environmental cues or owner behaviour, not their own behaviour whilst the owner was away. In one study owners were asked to shred some paper and then leave their dogs alone with it. On their return the dogs were reported to show appeasing behaviour, regardless of the fact they had not caused the damage.

In a more recent study dogs were trained to leave a treat when told and were then told to leave a treat whilst the owner left the room. The researcher stayed in the room and, once the owner had gone, either immediately removed the treat or encouraged the dog to eat it. When the owner then came back the researcher told some owners that their dog had eaten the treat and others they had not, regardless of what the dog had actually done. Those dogs whose owners thought they had stolen the treat appeased, regardless of what had actually happened, whereas if the owner thought they had not stolen it the dog did not appease. They also tried telling the dog to leave the treat then leaving the room until the dog finally stole it. Again, those dogs belonging to owners who were told the dog had stolen the treat showed appeasing but those who were told the dog had not stolen it did not, even though this time they actually had.

The head turning, avoidance of eye contact and withdrawal are therefore in response to the owner's annoyance, even if this is only mild, or other things in the environment they have learnt in the past trigger a punishment. It is not due to any sense of guilt or knowing they have done something wrong.

---

or wall, repetitive and purposeless vocalizations that lack interaction with the environment or compulsions linked to eating and drinking.

Compulsive behaviours develop when an animal is experiencing some kind of unpleasant emotion. They are therefore a sign of an underlying problem. Common triggers are summarized in Table 23.

Compulsive behaviours can be argued to be adaptive as they serve the purpose of redirecting emotions or fulfilling drives, enabling the animal to cope with less than ideal conditions. However, whilst not wholly abnormal they are dysfunctional in that they are a waste of an animal's resources. In severe cases they may also interfere with normal functioning such as eating, rest and social interaction, cause injury or put the animal at unnecessary risk.

Compulsive behaviours alleviate negative emotions by releasing exogenous endorphins. This can

Table 23. Common triggers for compulsive behaviour.

Trigger	Discussion
Frustration	This typically occurs when an animal is unable to fulfil a natural drive or achieve a reward for a prolonged period of time. Examples include dogs that spend a large amount of time confined, such as in a crate, dogs that have a strong drive to perform a behaviour which is frustrated or when rewards are withheld.
Deprivation or maltreatment	Such as if the dog is malnourishment or not being given sufficient companionship.
Emotional conflict	This occurs if the dog has two conflicting emotions that cannot be resolved, such as a strong drive to perform a behaviour and to avoid a punishment that has become associated to it.
Disease	Some diseases may cause compulsive behaviour, e.g. hepatic encephalopathy.
Inappropriate punishment	Where the punishment is excessive and/or the dog does not know how to prevent it.

then become self-rewarding over time. Therefore, some compulsive behaviour may persist even where the underlying problem has been corrected. This is especially so in breeds with enhanced internal reward systems, e.g. border collies and some terrier breeds. Compulsive behaviours can also become an effective attention seeking strategy.

Compulsive behaviours are not referred to as obsessive or an obsession in animals as the term obsession refers to repetitive thoughts. This cannot currently be measured in animals and so the term is best avoided.

Displacement activities

Displacement activities are behaviours performed to alleviate frustration at an inability to perform a desired behaviour. For example, an animal that paces when it cannot fulfil its demand for attention from its owner. This differs from compulsive behaviours purely in the lack of repetition.

Redirected behaviour

Redirected behaviour is the performance of a desired behaviour, but redirected to a secondary target. An example is where a dog that wants to threaten a person seen as invading its territory is unable to reach that person and so 'redirects' the behaviour on to another, e.g. the owner or another dog in the room.

Self-injurious behaviour

Self-injurious behaviour may take many guises such as over-grooming or tail biting and its causes can be multifactorial. However, where it does not have a physical cause it is generally accepted as an indicator of chronic stress and so a threat to welfare. It may or may not be stereotypic/compulsive.

Unwanted or Faulty Learning

Learning has a significant impact on the development of behaviour. Learning may occur intentionally or unintentionally and the dog may just as easily learn an unwanted as a wanted behaviour.

Intrinsic rewards

The learning of unwanted behaviours most frequently arises when the behaviour has an intrinsic reward. For example, a dog may learn that being able to open a fridge door will enable him to get to food. Alternatively he may learn that barking when shut in another room results in being let out. As such, owners need to try to put themselves in their dog's position so they can see what result the dog obtains from the unwanted behaviour. They can then ensure this is not inadvertently encouraging the dog to repeat it. This is discussed more in Chapter 7.

Issues with training

Learning of unwanted behaviour may also occur when attempts at training go wrong. For example, an owner may be intending to teach their dog not to urinate in the house by rubbing the dog's nose in the puddle when they find it, However, because there is such a long gap between the dog urinating and the owner finding it, the lesson the dog will have actually learnt is not to be around the owner when there is urine on the floor. This will then lead to the dog hiding from the owner when he next wants to urinate.

Another example is where a dog is asked to 'sit' after he has come back to the owner when called, before being given the treat. This rewards the dog for sitting but does not reward the recall. This may lead to continued failure to come when called.

Unwanted learning may also occur when dogs learn that aggression is effective and use it more frequently. This is particularly likely when dogs go through a pubescent period of 'testing boundaries' in adolescence.

7 Methods for Changing Behaviour

There are a number of ways in which we can change an animal's behaviour. Each has its own advantages and disadvantages and can be delivered in many different ways. It is therefore essential that a full history is taken, the cause of the problem behaviour is diagnosed and an understanding of the individual dog's character is determined before treatment is advised. Treatment delivery, whether by the professional or by the owner under the professional's guidance, also requires an understanding of how the treatment works and experience of its practical application. It is therefore a specialist area in all but the simplest of situations.

However, an awareness of the range of methods available will enable practice staff to inform clients of the type of help available, will help with delivery of prophylactic training and may enable practice staff to offer guidance for straightforward problems in house.

Conditioning

Classical and operant conditioning were briefly mentioned as part of how learning affects behaviour in Chapters 2 and 6. Their use in changing behaviour is skilled and requires the experience to manipulate the conditioning according to the individual dog's needs. What follows is therefore purely an introduction to the basic principles of using conditioning to manage or change behaviour.

Common principles of conditioning

Conditioning as a form of learning is occurring naturally all the time and unwanted or faulty conditioning is a common reason for the development of problem behaviour. It is also one of the easiest forms of learning to manipulate and so forms the basis for many behaviour modification plans.

Classical conditioning

At its simplest, learning by classical conditioning occurs when a naturally occurring involuntary physiological response becomes subconsciously linked to a previously unconnected external trigger. The new trigger then starts to elicit the original response on its own.

The classic example of this comes from Ivan Pavlov's research into the digestive system of dogs. Pavlov had inserted tubes into the salivary glands of dogs to measure the levels of saliva they produced as a natural response to being given meat powder. In classical conditioning the meat powder is an 'unconditioned stimulus' as it triggers salivation without the need for any form of conditioning. The salivation is an 'unconditioned response', because it again occurs without the need for conditioning.

As his research progressed Pavlov noticed the dogs were salivating before they were aware of the meat powder. He was not sure exactly what was causing this but realized that something in the process by which the food was being delivered must be acting as a signal of the food's arrival, which then caused the dogs to salivate. He therefore tried pairing ringing a bell with delivery of the meat powder to see what effect this had. At this stage the bell is described as a 'neutral' stimulus, i.e. it does not trigger the response of salivation naturally, nor has it yet become conditioned to it. By repeatedly pairing the bell and presentation of the meat powder he found that the bell alone started to trigger salivation. The bell then became a 'conditioned stimulus', i.e. even though a bell would not normally trigger salivation it will do once it has been conditioned to do so. The salivation became a 'conditioned response' as it was then happening in response to its conditioned link to the bell rather than as a natural response to the meat powder. This effect is depicted in Fig. 39.

Classical conditioning itself is a fairly simple principle. However, there are many factors that

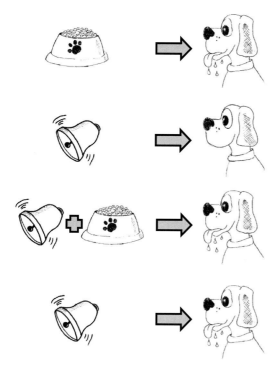

Fig. 39. Principles of classical conditioning.

influence whether it occurs and, if so, how strong the association. The key influences are as follows.

The saliency of the stimulus

Saliency refers to the relevance of the stimulus to the animal. Stimuli that hold little value are less likely to become classically conditioned to involuntary responses. For example, the ticking of a clock is unlikely to become conditioned if the animal has habituated to it, as he will not be taking any notice of it. However, if the clock has a chime, or if it is a new clock with a very loud or different tick this may be more noticeable to the dog and so may be conditioned. If the dog is always fed when the clock chimes five times this will further intensify its relevance to the dog and so conditioning.

Overshadowing and blocking

If there are two stimuli one may 'overshadow' or 'block' the other. In overshadowing the dog forms a stronger association to a more noticeable or salient stimulus than to a lesser one. For example, if

both a bright blue light and a dim white light are flashed when a dog is presented with food then he will make a stronger association to the blue light than the white one. In blocking a stimulus the dog is already conditioned to block any association forming with a new stimulus. So if the dog is first conditioned to salivate in response to a blue light, he won't then condition to a white light despite its being paired with food.

Timing

The order in which the neutral and the unconditioned stimulus occur in relation to each other can affect how strong the conditioning is. Classical conditioning occurs due to the dog learning that the neutral stimulus (bell) predicts the unconditioned stimulus (food). Conditioning is therefore strongest if the neutral stimulus (bell) starts before the unconditioned stimulus (food) appears. Conditioning is less strong if the neutral and unconditioned stimulus both start and end together and is weakest if the unconditioned stimulus (food) starts and ends before the neutral stimulus (bell) occurs (see Fig. 40).

Consistency

Pairings need to be consistently repeated for the association to be made. They also need to be maintained or the pairing will break down (referred to as extinction – see below).

Systematic desensitization and counter-conditioning

Sensitization occurs where the dog has developed an increased sensitivity and so reaction to a stimulus after repeated exposure. This can involve any response, but in dogs it is most typically due to either fear or excitement and their associated behaviours. In the case of fear it may occur due to one severely unpleasant or numerous moderately unpleasant experiences around the stimulus. These may be genuinely unpleasant experiences or ones that dogs perceive as such, e.g. due to poor coping ability. Desensitization is the process whereby this sensitization is broken down.

The aim of desensitization is to expose the dog to the stimulus in a controlled way so that he habituates to it. The animal's reaction then changes

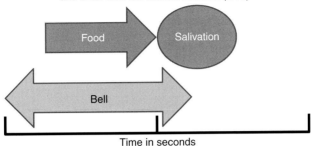

Delay timing – most effective

The stimulus to be conditioned (bell) starts before
and ends after the natural stimulus (food)

Food

Salivation

Bell

Time in seconds

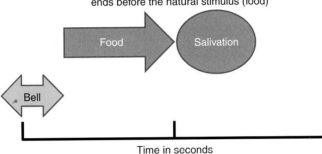

Trace timing – moderately effective

The stimulus to be conditioned (bell) starts and
ends before the natural stimulus (food)

Food

Salivation

Bell

Time in seconds

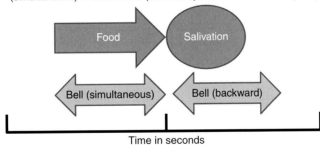

Simultaneous or Backward timing – poor efficacy

The stimulus to be conditioned (bell) starts and ends with
(simultaneous) or starts after (backward) the natural stimulus (food)

Food

Salivation

Bell (simultaneous)

Bell (backward)

Time in seconds

Fig. 40. Effects of timing in classical conditioning.

from negative (e.g. fearful) to neutral (i.e. indifferent) (see Fig. 41).

Counter-conditioning is the process whereby the dog's current emotional response is replaced by another, more positive one. Changes to the current emotional state occur by classically conditioning a new emotional response to the stimulus currently triggering an unwanted emotion (see Fig. 41). For example, fear can be replaced with the pleasure derived from food, play or affection. Desensitization is usually needed before counter-conditioning. This is because in many cases the level of fear prior to

Methods for Changing Behaviour

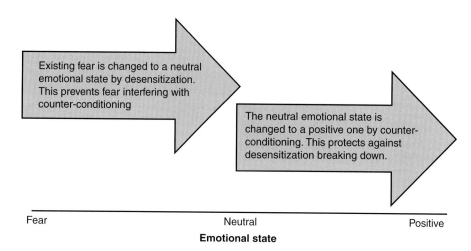

Fear   Neutral   Positive

Emotional state

Fig. 41. Emotional changes that occur during desensitization and classical counter-conditioning.

treatment is too high for the dog to be able to play games or accept food. However, once the dog has desensitized to the trigger the fear is then low enough for counter-conditioning to start. Counter-conditioning is needed after desensitization as the neutral response triggered by the latter is very susceptible to breaking down. Counter- conditioning a positive emotional response significantly lessens the likelihood of this.

Desensitization and counter-conditioning do not erase the previously conditioned response. They rely instead on the newly conditioned response being stronger and therefore preferable to the old one. It will therefore require time and commitment to ensure that the associations made during the programme are more intense and more numerous than the associations made during the development of the unwanted behaviour. This is one of the reasons why early treatment is so important.

When performing this type of training it is important to control the level of exposure. If the exposure is too strong the stress it causes may block the dog's ability to learn the stimulus is not harmful. However, the dog must be aware of it for the conditioning to work. The practitioner must therefore aim to set the initial intensity of the stimulus at the point at which the dog is first aware of it, but below the point at which he is concerned by it. How to do this depends on the nature of the trigger.

If the trigger is a tangible object (e.g. a dog, passing cars) distance will reduce intensity in most cases. Typically each dog will have a distance at which they do not react to or even notice the trigger at all. At a

closer distance they will be aware of the trigger but their level of fear will be low. As they get gradually closer the intensity of the fear will rise until it is intense enough to trigger a reaction. The dog's level of awareness and fear can be determined by watching their behaviour for signs of vigilance to the trigger or early signs of stress. Maximum success is achieved by keeping the dog at the distance at which he is just aware of but not noticeably fearful of it. An example is given in Fig. 42 and the key steps in a programme of desensitization and counter-conditioning are outlined in Box 7.1.

Programmes of desensitization and counter-conditioning need to be performed carefully and require experience to judge the triggers, how to control them and to read the dog's response to them. They are therefore best conducted by a specialist in this area. However, simple programmes that may be able to be followed by the veterinary team are discussed in Chapter 14.

Operant conditioning

Operant conditioning is the process whereby an animal modifies voluntary behaviours according to their learnt outcome. If they learn the behaviour has a good outcome they will repeat it. If they learn the behaviour has a bad outcome they will avoid repeating it.

Operant conditioning occurs naturally through 'trial and error'. A dog will try a behaviour to see if it obtains the desired outcome. The desired outcome may be for something good to happen (e.g. to get some

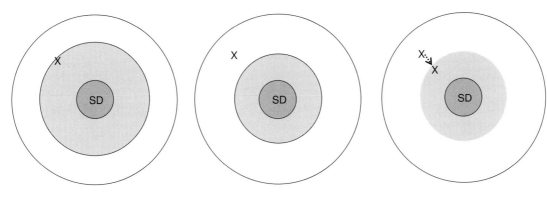

Training starts at the distance at which the dog is aware of the other dog but is not worried by it.

After training the dog will stop attending to the trigger at this distance.

The dog can then move a little closer.

X   The dog being trained
SD The 'stooge' dog

At this distance the dog is not interested in the trigger

At this distance the dog is attending to but not showing higher levels of fear to the trigger

At this distance the dog will show and feel higher level fear

The precise way the distance at which training starts and progresses is determined depends on the trigger, the individual dog and the circumstances. In this example the dog's desire to look at the other dog is used to indicate a very low level of concern and so the right distance at which to conduct the training. If the dog was so far away from the stooge dog that he showed no interest at all this would indicate he is either not aware of or not at all concerned by other dogs at that distance and so the training would not change anything. If he was close enough to show more marked signs of fear then this may get in the way of the training. It would also raise ethical questions for the dog, and the stooge if the fear was being shown as threat. The balance is therefore keeping the dog where he is aware of but not scared by the other dog. Once he no longer shows signs of wanting to pay attention to the other dog at all this suggests he now feels no concern at this new distance. He can then be moved closer.

Fig. 42. Controlling the intensity of the trigger in desensitization and classical counter-conditioning.

Box 7.1. The key steps in a programme of desensitization and classical counter-conditioning.

- Minimize exposure to the trigger other than for training to prevent further sensitization.
- Control other negative stimuli during training.
- Determine at what level the dog attends to but is not fearful of the trigger.
- Expose the animal to this level of intensity.
- Maintain exposure until the dog no longer attends to the stimulus.

- Perform activities to evoke pleasure, e.g. feeding, playing, training etc., according to the dog's individual needs.
- Repeat until the dog can cope with this level of stimulus quickly and easily.
- Increase intensity and repeat.
- If at any stage the dog shows higher level fear stop and go back a step. Allow him to perform normal coping mechanisms.

---

food) or may be for something bad to stop (avoid being smacked). If the behaviour gets the desired outcome the dog will repeat it. If it does not they may repeat it a few more times, then try something else. If it gets an unpleasant outcome, such as leading to being smacked or failing to stop them from being smacked, they will avoid doing it again. They will try something else instead.

For example, if a dog wants some food that has been left on a table they may first try putting their paws on the table to see if they can steal the food. If they manage to get the food this way they may do this again next time there is food left out. However, if, after a few repetitions, they are unable to get the food this way they may try something else, e.g. getting on a chair. If this works they will choose this way first next time. Alternatively if putting their paws on the table causes something to fall on to their head they may avoid doing so in the future. However, that does not mean they will not still try to get the food – they will just try a different way. If trying another way also causes things to fall on their head they may stop that too, but will often still try other methods until they run out of things to try or are no longer motivated to do so.

Although the majority of operant conditioning arises naturally, people can also use this method of learning to manipulate an animal's behaviour. Most forms of animal training rely on giving the animal a reward when they perform a desired behaviour and punishing the animal when unwanted behaviour occurs (the precise definition of punishment will be discussed further below). Behaviour modification also often relies on rewarding wanted and 'punishing' unwanted behaviours to change whichever behaviour the dog chooses to perform.

Rewards and punishments in operant conditioning

Rewards and punishments form an intrinsic part of training using operant conditioning. However, the terms can be confusing, partly because they have colloquial as well as scientific meanings and also because so many different terms are used to describe them.

In operant conditioning a reward is something that increases repetition of the behaviour the dog sees as having triggered the reward. This can occur by giving the dog something he wants or by stopping something he does not want at the time he performs the behaviour to be encouraged. Rewards are also called 'appetitives' or 'reinforcers'. The term reward will be used for simplicity.

In operant conditioning a punishment is something that decreases the repetition of the behaviour the dog links it to. This can occur by applying something the dog does not want or by taking something he does want away when he performs the behaviour to be deterred. Punishments are also called 'aversives'. The term punishment will be used.

One way to illustrate how rewards and punishments work is by placing the four ways these can be delivered in a table (see Table 24). This shows how rewards can increase behaviours by adding something the dog wants or taking away something they do not want, and punishments can decrease repetition of behaviour by doing the opposite. The implications of each of the quadrants are discussed more below.

Both rewards and punishments only work if they are delivered correctly. This means they must be delivered consistently, at the right time and at the right intensity.

Timing

Correct timing is essential if the animal is to understand which behaviour the person is trying to reward or punish. To be effective the reward or punishment must be given as the animal is performing the behaviour it is intended to influence. If it is given at any other time the animal will associate the outcome with whatever he is doing at that time. For example, if a dog urinates on the kitchen floor when his owner is out and the owner then comes home and punishes him for doing so

Table 24. Rewards and punishments in operant conditioning.

	Reward *Increases repetition of the* *linked behaviour*	Punishment *Decreases repetition of the* *linked behaviour*
Positive *Adding something*	*Add something desirable* Give the dog something that evokes pleasure, e.g. food, play or attention	*Add something undesirable* Apply something that causes fear or pain, e.g. physical punishment, check chains, electric shocks or fear-inducing noises
Negative *Taking something away*	*Take away something undesirable* Stop applying the stimulus that causes fear or pain, e.g. physical punishment, check chains, electric shocks or fear-inducing noises	*Take away something desirable* Stop giving the dog the thing that evokes pleasure, e.g. food, play or attention

the dog will associate the punishment with the owner's arrival, not the urination.

Consistency

The outcome must be applied consistently. If the outcome is only given some of the times the animal performs the behaviour it will take much longer for the dog to make the association. Inconsistency can also affect motivation. For example, if an owner tries to encourage their dog to go to his bed when visitors arrive but only occasionally rewards him for doing so then the reward offered for obeying might be outweighed by the intrinsic reward the dog gets from greeting the visitors (see below regarding schedules of rewards).

Intensity and saliency

The intensity and saliency of the outcome must be appropriate for it to be effective in modifying behaviour. If a reward is small or something the dog does not value then the motivation to repeat the behaviour to get it is lessened. Equally, if the positive reward is too big the dog may quickly tire of it, after which the value of the reward will lessen. In the same way, if a positive punishment is too mild or something the dog does not see as unpleasant his motivation to avoid repeating the behaviour will be reduced. However, if it is too strong the stress triggered may interfere with

his ability to learn. This will be discussed in more detail below. Additional factors affecting the saliency of rewards and punishments are outlined in Table 25.

Conditioned 'outcomes'

Training with operant conditioning usually involves direct and immediate delivery of the reward or punishment. However, this may sometimes be problematic. This can be overcome by using a stimulus that has been conditioned to a reward or punishment. This stimulus can then be used to communicate to the dog what they are being rewarded or punished for. The types of stimuli that can be employed are summarized in Table 26.

Associations are made by repeatedly pairing the stimulus to be conditioned and the outcome to which it is to be linked. For example, a clicker (Fig. 43) is typically conditioned to a positive reward by repeatedly clicking and then giving the dog a treat. Equally 'training discs' (Fig. 44) can be conditioned as a negative punishment by placing a treat on the floor and then rattling the discs and removing the treat when the dog tries to take it.

One of the key advantages of using these markers is improved timing. The stimuli used for conditioned rewards and punishments are typically very brief. They are therefore able to be given exactly as the behaviour to be influenced occurs. This can

Table 25. Factors affecting the saliency of rewards and punishments.

Factor	Description
Intrinsic outcome	The intensity of the reward or punishment delivered has to compete with the intrinsic reward that comes from the behaviour the dog would choose for himself. For example, the reward for not stealing or punishment for stealing food needs to outweigh the intrinsic reward attained by doing so.
Availability and repeated use	Rewards that are freely available hold lower value than those that are not. Only allowing access to highly valued rewards to when training maintains their value. Dogs may also desensitize to punishments that are used frequently especially milder ones.
Arousal level	The more aroused a dog is, whether by fear or excitement, the less focused he will be on the reward or punishment. Its intensity therefore needs to be greater to have the desired effect. This is normally addressed by lowering the excitement/fear rather than increasing the reward/punishment, but it is important to be aware of this effect.
Individual variation	The value each dog places on a reward or punishment will vary. This may be influenced by breed, past experiences and individual variation. For example, labradors are commonly food motivated whereas border collies are highly rewarded by balls/chasing. However, a labrador that has been trained to enjoy retrieving will also be driven by balls.

Table 26. Common items used to condition a reward or punishment in operant conditioning.

Conditioned Outcome	Description
Clickers	A device that makes a clicking noise (see Fig. 43).
Training discs	A fabric ring containing four or five small metal cymbals that make a distinctive sound when rattled together (see Fig. 44).
Verbal rewards or punishments	Words can become conditioned to an outcome, e.g. 'good boy', 'uh-oh'.
Human non-lexical signals	Any sound a human can make can be conditioned if it is noticeable to the animal, e.g. a 'tut tut' or raspberry.

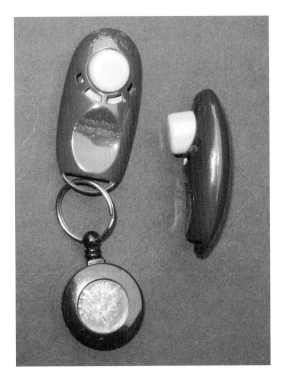

Fig. 43. A clicker.

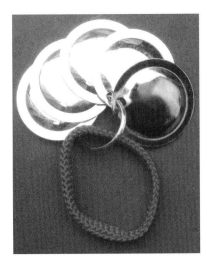

Fig. 44. Training discs.

Training schedules

The dog will only initially make an association between a behaviour and a reward or punishment if the same outcome occurs every time the dog performs the behaviour. The outcome needs to be maintained permanently when using positive punishment, otherwise the dog's original drive to perform the unwanted behaviour will resurface. Inconsistent delivery of positive punishers also carries the risk of triggering anxiety or aggression (see below). However, when using positive reward it is possible to reduce their frequency once the behaviour is established. The frequency with which rewards can be delivered is discussed in Table 27.

Although continuous reward schedules give the dog a reliable outcome for their behaviour and help the behaviour initially become established, the behaviour tends to stop very quickly if the delivery of the rewards stops and the dog will often only perform the behaviour if they can see the food.

improve the dog's understanding of which behaviour triggered the outcome. Timing is also improved by the fact they can be used from a distance. For example, if a dog performs a behaviour the owner wants to encourage when on the other side of the room it is impossible to give the reward quickly enough for the dog to make a clear association. However, the delay between the behaviour and the reward can be 'bridged' by giving the conditioned outcome as the behaviour occurs and then going to the dog or calling him to you for the reward. There may be a delay but the marker will have told the dog what the reward is for.

Moving on to a fixed or variable schedule can perversely improve the reliability with which the dog will perform the behaviour that is rewarded.

Using a fixed schedule teaches the dog they will have to repeat the behaviour multiple times before they get any reward. The intervals have to be built up very gradually whilst the dog learns there is now a delay in the delivery of the reward. There is also a risk that the reliability of the behaviour may reduce immediately following the reward as the dog realizes the next one is a long way off.

Variable schedules make the reward unpredictable. The dog therefore never knows when it is next coming. This prevents the sudden cessation that occurs in continuous schedules and the reduction in reliability of the behaviour associated with fixed intervals, because the dog anticipates the reward may come at any time. The intervals have to be built up gradually as above.

Using trained commands to change behaviour

The most common way of using conditioning to manage or change behaviour with dogs is to train them to respond to 'commands' or 'cues'. The cue is most commonly either a word or other auditory signal such as a whistle, or a visual hand signal. However, any of the senses can be employed and imaginative cues can be employed with dogs with sensory impairment, e.g. lights, touches or true vibration (not shock) collars in deaf dogs (see Chapter 12). The association between the cue, the behaviour and the desired outcome is most simply achieved by using food or another desirable stimulus to lure the behaviour, then giving the cue (to make the association) and delivering the positive reward. Once the association has been repeated a number of times the cue may be given without the lure and the behaviour rewarded if it occurs. More complex or subtle behaviours can be taught using a variety of methods described in Table 28.

Trained commands can be used to manage or manipulate the dog to voluntarily follow owner's wishes, either temporarily or permanently according to the situation. For example, if a dog barks when the doorbell rings this can be managed by teaching him to go to a 'mat' on command. Giving a pre-emptive command can also be used to prevent predictably undesirable behaviour. This both manages it and

Table 27. Reward schedules used in operant conditioning.

Schedule	Discussion
Continuous reward schedule	The reward is given every time the behaviour occurs. This is required initially to enable associations to be made.
Fixed reward schedule	The reward can be given at fixed time intervals, e.g. every 5 s regardless of how many repetitions of the behaviour have occurred, providing they have occurred consistently. Alternatively they can be given after a fixed number of repetitions of the behaviour e.g. every five times.
Variable reward schedule	The reward can be given at variable time intervals, e.g. after 5 s, then after 3 s, then after 7 s regardless of how many repetitions of the behaviour have occurred, providing they have occurred consistently. Alternatively they can be given after a variable number of repetitions e.g. after 5 times, then 3 times, then 7 times.

Table 28. Operant conditioning techniques used to teach advanced behaviours.

Method	Description
Chaining	Multiple behaviours are trained and then linked together.
Shaping	Complex, precise or difficult to lure behaviours can be taught by initially teaching a behaviour similar to the one required and then gradually only rewarding a behaviour that is slightly closer until the desired behaviour is reached.
Targeting	A target stick or similar object is used to lure the animal to perform required behaviours, which can then be named and/or rewarded or shaped.
Fading	Once a task has been trained the signals or cues used to lure the behaviour can be gradually reduced until they are almost imperceptible.

changes the dog's habitual behaviour in that situation. Alternatively the dog can be requested to do something that prevents the unwanted behaviour, e.g. asking a dog that jumps up to 'sit'. Finally the behaviour can be 'put on cue'. If a dog is taught to perform unwanted behaviour on command it then becomes easier to control the behaviour or teach a counter behaviour. For example, dogs that are taught to bark on command can then be taught to be 'quiet' on command too.

Using commands in this way tends to rely on rewarding the preferred behaviour and ensuring the intrinsic rewards for the unwanted behaviour are removed. For example, asking a dog to sit to be greeted and completely ignoring any jumping up, rewards sitting and uses negative punishment to deter jumping up as a way to get attention. When doing so the client must be made aware that there may be a transient increase in the unwanted behaviour before it finally stops altogether. This is referred to as an extinction burst. It occurs because the animal is becoming frustrated that the behaviour no longer elicits the reward it used to. They therefore try harder to get it. For example, jumping up behaviour that is being ignored can get more intense before it subsides. This is the point at which many owners give up in the belief the treatment is making things worse not better. However, it is actually a sign the dog has noticed the behaviour no longer gets the desired response and so a sign that it *is* working.

Positive, reward or force-free training

'Positive', 'reward based' and 'force free' are the colloquial terms used to describe trainers who utilize operant conditioning by adding a reward for wanted behaviour and withholding it for unwanted behaviour.

The criticism typically levied at positive trainers is that they leave unwanted behaviour uncorrected and that some behaviour cannot be changed purely by giving or withholding desirable things such as treats. However, this argument fails to recognize the consequences imposed for unwanted behaviour by withholding what the dog wants. If done skilfully this can be very powerful.

Changing what the dog wants to do by manipulating rewards for desired behaviour is also recognized as having a longer term effect than punishing behaviour does. If the outcome of a behaviour is something the dog finds unpleasant he will avoid repeating the behaviour. However, this does not change the dog's desire to achieve the original aim, e.g. to steal the food. The dog will therefore try again another way or on another day. Permanent change only occurs where the dog's desire to perform the behaviour has been changed, or they have learned a better way to get what they want.

Positive punishment or 'balanced' training

'Punishment' training is the colloquial term used to describe trainers or behaviourists that utilize operant conditioning by adding a punishment for unwanted behaviour and stopping it once the desired behaviour is performed. 'Balanced training' is often used to describe trainers that use a combination of all four options depending on the situation. For example, they may use the 'positive reward' of giving a treat if a dog sits when asked, and the 'negative punishment' of withholding it when they do not, mixed with the 'positive punishment' of an electric shock if the dog will not come when called and the 'negative reward' of ending the shock when the dog comes back.

The effects of fear and pain on learning

It is important to understand properly how dogs react to fear and pain in order to be able to objectively evaluate the risks and benefits of using positive punishment.

Initial exposure to a fearful stimulus sends messages to the amygdala, part of the brain responsible for the regulation of emotions and memory formation, to stimulate the 'fight or flight' response. This results in physiological changes that enable and drive the dog to take steps to increase his distance from the trigger, either by withdrawing or by using threat. The intrinsically unpleasant sensations of fear also drive the animal to repel or avoid the trigger, or any other stimulus that becomes classically conditioned to it, on subsequent occasions. This occurs through operant conditioning, i.e. the dog learns that being close to the trigger or a classically associated trigger leads to the unwanted outcome of feeling unpleasantly fearful and so avoids doing so in the future. This is a survival mechanism that helps the dog avoid potentially dangerous situations.

The sensation of physical pain is one of the body's responses to stimulation of specialized sensory neurons (nociceptors) by noxious stimuli. Pain can be triggered by physical stretching or bending of nociceptors, application of excessive heat or cold, oxygen deprivation causing lactic acid production or tissue damage from chemicals. Once stimulated nociceptor messages transcend the spinal column to the brain where they are registered and trigger the autonomic system to respond. This may include activating the limbic system, causing fear, the association cortices to generate learned associations and the fight or flight centres to trigger an acute stress or defensive response. This may in turn lead to a chronic stress response dependent on the situation.

The immediate voluntary response to pain is usually termination of the behaviour seen to have triggered it, although this will be balanced between the degree of pain and the intrinsic reward from the behaviour. If the dog learns to expect pain as a consequence for certain behaviours changes in the association cortex lower the likelihood the behaviour will be repeated (subject to below).

A dog's perception of pain is highly subjective and can be influenced by many factors. A chronically anxious animal is more likely to react to pain whereas a highly aroused or chronically stressed animal is less likely to. The presence of endogenous opiates, analgesic pharmaceuticals and sensitization or habituation due to previous use of punishments will affect perception of pain. Perception can also be affected by factors such as coat and skin thickness.

Methods of positive punishment

Positive punishment may be delivered in many ways. The key methods are summarized in Box 7.2.

Direct physical punishment describes any technique that creates an impact on any part of the dog's body, using a part of the human body or an

---

> **Box 7.2. Summary of methods of applying positive punishments.**
>
> - Direct physical punishment.
> - Intimidation.
> - Forced manipulation.
> - Check or slip collars and leads.
> - Dominant Dog™, Snap Around or Volhard collar.
> - Half-check collars.
> - Prong or pinch collars.
> - Static pulse, electric shock, 'stim' or E collars.
> - Vapour or gas training collars.
> - Sonic devices.
> - Air canisters.
> - Rattle devices.

---

implement. Human contact typically involves using the hand, foot or two rigidly held fingers to make contact with part of the dog's body such as the back of the neck, the rump, the thigh or the underside of the neck or belly. Implements commonly used include leads, chains and rolled up newspapers.

Some who use these techniques suggest they are used in a way that correct behaviour without being punishing to the dog. If the contact is light enough to not be unpleasant the dog may just ignore it, especially if he is aroused or performing a behaviour he enjoys. Alternatively it may draw his attention away from the trigger and on to the person making the contact. In this case the handler will then need to give another command or perform another action to direct the dog's behaviour. If they do not the dog will be distracted momentarily but the behaviour will not be changed. He is then very likely to go back to what he was doing before and will probably quickly learn to ignore this type of contact from the owner as being irrelevant. As such the principles of operant conditioning dictate that if the contact is intended to or is effective in changing the behaviour it will need to or is being given with sufficient force to be aversive to the dog.

Intimidation involves behaviour or postures that imply the person will cause the dog harm such as by staring at or standing over the dog in a threatening manner. Dominance hierarchy theorists often suggest them as a way to assert the human role as 'pack leader'. The threat involved may inhibit behaviour through operant positive punishment, i.e. fear. It may also make the dog chronically fearful of the person delivering the 'threat' or may lead to defensive aggression at the time or on subsequent occasions.

Methods of forced manipulation include forcibly preventing or making the dog perform a required behaviour, pushing the dog against a solid object (e.g. wall) or forcing the dog on to its side or back. In most cases these methods evoke fear through intimidation rather than pain, although the latter is possible depending on the degree of force used. Rolling the dog on to its back is suggested to mimic how a wolf would correct a subordinate pack member that is challenging it. As the dog is not a wolf, how wolves behave is not relevant. Dogs do not ordinarily force other dogs on to their backs. It may occur rarely as misdirected predatory behaviour or in extreme cases of heightened aggression. However, if one dog ends up on his back during an interaction with another dog he has usually arrived there as a voluntary act of appeasement. Therefore

---

if a human pushes a dog on to his back the dog will see this as highly threatening, resulting in very high levels of fear and possible defensive aggression. It is also common for this type of correction to be the trigger for the dog using higher levels of aggression on subsequent interactions with people due to the anticipation this may happen again.

Check and slip collars and leads form a moving loop around the dog's neck that can be tightened or loosened by the handler (see Figs 45 and 46). They are typically made from chain or rope. Chain devices normally involve just a collar to which a separate lead is attached. Rope devices may be either a collar with a separate lead attached or a single length of rope to serve as both. The 'Snap-Around Training Collar' (also called the Volhard collar) and the Dominant Dog Collar™ are variations of a slip collar, in which the collar is sized to fit snugly around the dog's neck behind the ears so it will not slip down. The rope versions are also sometimes looped over the nose to create a pseudo-head collar

(see Fig. 47). This reduces the constriction around the neck but has been known to cause significant skin and soft tissue abrasion through rubbing. Most variations are intended to deter pulling by briefly tightening and then releasing the collar or lead when the dog is in the incorrect position. The constriction triggers pain or fear of asphyxiation. It is currently popular to recommend the collar is placed as high on the neck as possible, which intensifies this effect (see Fig. 48). Efficacy is determined by the degree of pain or fear used versus the dog's drive to pull. Some dogs quickly habituate to the discomfort and routinely pull against it, often choking themselves to the point of noticeable hypoxia. Others may only pull when highly aroused, such as dogs that show high-level defensive aggression. In this case the fear drives the dog to persist with pulling despite the pain or reduced blood and so oxygen supply to the head. Rarely trainers may advocate suspending the dog via the collar/lead as a more advanced aversive. These devices carry significant risks and have been linked to orthopaedic, soft tissue and brain damage and have been responsible for deaths in dogs (e.g. Grohmann *et al.*, 2013). This can occur even if the dog is applying the higher pressure himself by pulling if the fight or flight response is overriding their need to avoid self-asphyxiation.

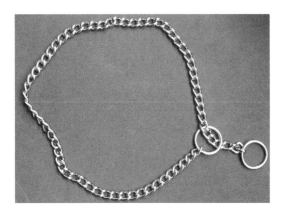

Fig. 45. Check chain.

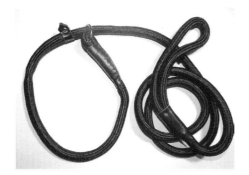

Fig. 46. Slip lead.

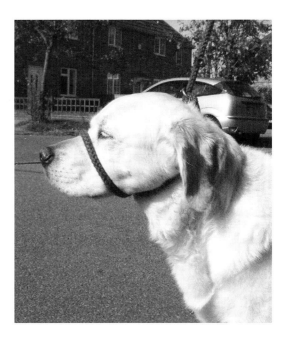

Fig. 47. Slip lead used as a head collar.

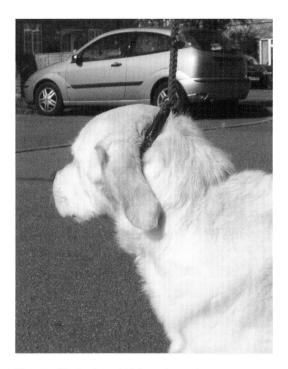

Fig. 48. Slip lead used high on the neck.

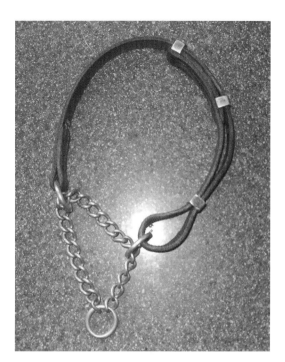

Fig. 49. Half-check collar.

Half-check collars incorporate a loop of chain into a flat cloth or leather collar to which the lead is attached (see Fig. 49). Tightening of the chain constricts the collar around the dog's neck. However, this is limited according to how tightly the collar is fitted. They therefore range from as aversive as a check chain to not aversive at all, depending on fit.

Prong or pinch collars have inward facing curved spikes (see Fig. 50). Tightening of the collar is controlled by a loop of chain to which the lead is attached, as with half-check collars. The degree of adversity (i.e. the degree to which the prongs dig into the dog's neck) therefore varies according to fitting, although all will cause some distress even with normal wear. Excessively tight collars can cause severe skin and soft tissue damage. Patented designs may vary in principle but not in effect, e.g. the Pro-Training collar® (see Fig. 51). Their action is to increase the intensity of the pain achieved with a standard check collar through the points of the prongs. Some have suggested the prongs mimic a dog's bite but it is highly unlikely that a dog would mistake an inanimate object with metal prongs for another dog.

Static pulse (also referred to as electric shock, remote, 'stim' or E collars) apply a pulse of electricity via probes in contact with the dog's skin (see Figs 52 and 53). The intensity and duration of the shock can be varied on some models and some have a cut-out to prevent prolonged impulse delivery. Shocks can be delivered manually via a remote control. Alternatively they may be triggered automatically by sensors such as vibration sensors triggered by barking or barrier sensors that trigger a shock if the animal approaches a boundary. Some incorporate audio or visual 'warning' signals that the dog learns predict a shock if they do not stop the trigger behaviour. However, the dog still needs to receive the shock repeatedly to make the initial association. These should not be confused with true vibration collars that genuinely only vibrate and do not have prongs so are incapable of delivering an electrical impulse. Static pulse collars are illegal in Wales, UK and other countries. They carry all the risks associated with positive punishments discussed below. The collars that are triggered by sensor carry the greatest risks, closely followed by collars in the hands of unskilled trainers, due to the possibility of the dog making incorrect associations or the

Methods for Changing Behaviour

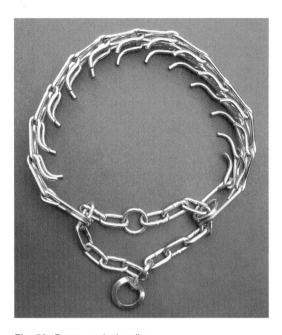

Fig. 50. Prong or pinch collar.

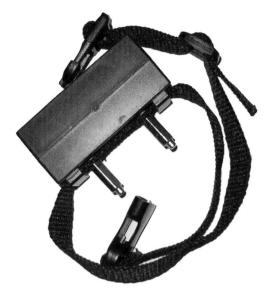

Fig. 52. Bark-activated static pulse, electric shock, remote, stim or E collar.

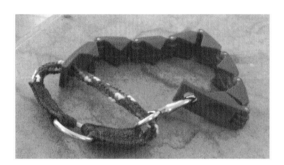

Fig. 51. Pro-Training collar®.

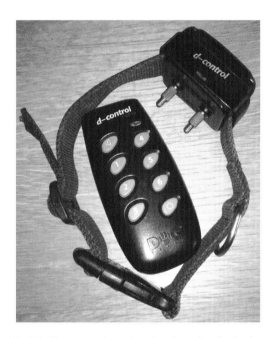

Fig. 53. Remote-activated static pulse, electric shock, remote, stim or E collar.

punishment being delivered in a way the dog finds unpredictable, leading to anxiety and defensive aggression (see below).

Vapour or gas training collars deliver citronella or water vapour, or inert gases (see Fig. 54). They are triggered by vibration (e.g. barking) or manually via a remote control. Sonic devices emit ultrasonic sounds via a unit which may be free standing or attached to a collar. They may be activated by vibration or sound (e.g. barking), or manually by remote control. Air canisters involve a canister of compressed gas, which is released manually close to the animal (see Fig. 55). They are suggested to signal danger in domestic pets, which will trigger

an instinctive fear response. Rattle devices refer to various methods of causing a sudden rattling sound close to the dog, e.g. cans or bottles of stones, chains (loose or in a bag), tin cans tied

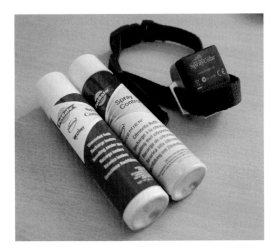

Fig. 54. Spray collar.

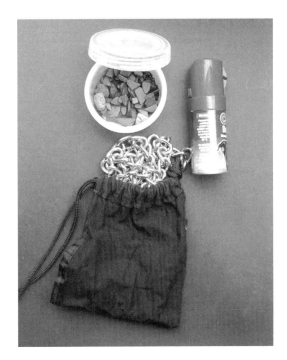

Fig. 55. Startle aversives including an air canister, rattle can and chain in a bag.

together or keys (see Fig. 55). Training discs can also be used in this way although that is not the manufacturer's intention. These are all 'startle' techniques. If the individual dog does not find the method used aversive the novelty of the noise may draw their attention and so interrupt the behaviour, allowing the handler to then direct a more suitable response. However, this effect tends to wear off after a few days or weeks in most dogs as they habituate to the noise. If the dog finds the noise genuinely aversive it then acts as a positive punishment. If the method is effective at changing a behaviour then it must be accepted the dog is seeing it as such.

Concerns with the use of positive punishment

Criticism of the use of positive punishments tends to focus on the welfare implications, efficacy and potential adverse effects. The welfare arguments are complex and in places subjective. To what degree the dog finds the applied aversive truly distressing is difficult to measure scientifically. There is evidence to show dogs trained using electronic training collars have heightened levels of stress hormones both at the time of training and in subsequent similar situations (Schilder and van der Borg, 2004; Schalke *et al.*, 2007). However, it can be argued that not all stress is bad and stress does not automatically imply negative emotions. Furthermore, even if it is accepted that the dog is in distress some will argue that it is justified if the positive punishment

saves the dog from being euthanized. The discussion regarding their use is therefore more objective if it focuses on whether the claim they are more effective than positive reward is true and so can be used to justify their use, and on the risks associated with them.

Studies comparing the efficacy of the two forms of conditioning consistently show that, providing it is delivered correctly, positive reward is at least as effective and often more so than positive punishment. For example, Hiby *et al.* (2004) found prevention of chewing, teaching a dog to walk to heel and to give up stolen items were all significantly more responsive to positive reward than positive punishment training. None of the behaviours they evaluated responded better to positive punishment methods than rewards. Blackwell *et al.* (2012) showed that more owners reported success with rewards than remote collar training for recall training and chase behaviour. Rooney and Cowan (2011) found dogs trained with positive rewards perform better on new tasks, suggesting an on-going effect on the dog's trainability according to method used (Cooper *et al.* (2013a). Positive punishment was also found to reduce activity, which in turn reduces opportunities for operant learning (Shors, 2004). As such there is no evidence to support the suggestion that positive punishment is more effective than positive reward.

Studies have also highlighted the risks associated with the use of positive punishment, both to animal welfare and owner safety. The need for the manipulated outcome to be accurately timed and consistently delivered for the dog to work out which behaviour led to the reward or punishment has been discussed above. Punishments that are not delivered consistently correctly therefore simply become random acts of aggression in the dog's eyes. This can result in fear of the person or chronic anxiety. This effect was demonstrated by Schalke et al. (2007) during a study in which shocks were given randomly to laboratory beagles to mimic poorly timed or inconsistent delivery of punishments. The dogs showed elevated levels of stress both at the time of training and when returning to the training centre 4 weeks later, demonstrating the potential chronic effects of poorly delivered punishments on animal welfare.

Even where punishments are correctly timed their intensity also needs to be correct to have the desired effect. Wells (2001) showed that dogs may quickly habituate to aversives they do not find strongly distressing, so they cease to be effective. Conversely, where the intensity of the punisher is too high this may trigger pain and/or fear, anxiety or chronic stress. Cooper et al. (2013b) found that 36% of dogs yelped on the first application of a shock collar by a positive punishment professional and 26% of dogs continued to do so on subsequent applications. The pain this indicates will have triggered associated stress and fear. Stress is known to interfere with memory formation and operant learning in some individuals (Cavanagh et al., 2011), therefore undermining the purpose of the punishment. Circulating cortisol levels were also seen when the same dogs were returned to the same training ground a few months later, even without use of the collar, suggesting the stress and so potential interference with learning is prolonged.

Punishments have also been shown to carry the risk of being associated with the owner rather than the behaviour as intended. Schilder and van der Borg (2004) found that dogs previously trained using shock collars showed greater physiological stress and fearful body language during subsequent training sessions with their handler, even where the shock collar was not put on.

Finally, punishments risk triggering a defensive response, either at the time of its delivery or on subsequent occasions. This principle was supported by Herron et al. (2009), who found that a substantial proportion of dogs reacted to confrontational or positive punishment-based corrections with immediate aggression (see Fig. 56). Dogs trained using positive punishment were also shown to be more likely to show defensive behaviour by Arhant et al. (2010).

Advocates of positive punishment claim it is sometimes justified as the only way to correct behaviour that will otherwise lead to relinquishment or euthanasia. However, independent evidence shows that positive punishment is no more and in many cases is less effective than positive reward even for highly self-rewarding behaviour such as chase and predation. That justification therefore cannot be upheld. Therefore, as precise delivery is challenging and incorrect use carries substantial risk of injury to the handler, and long-term undesirable and sometimes irreversible behaviour such as chronic fear of people, anxiety and pre-emptive defensive aggression there is no objective support for its use.

Response prevention (flooding)

Response prevention, also often referred to as flooding, is a controversial method of desensitization sometimes used in human psychology. It is based on the principle that avoidance of a trigger prevents habituation. The person or dog is exposed to the stimulus at its full intensity until the acute 'fight or flight' response is exhausted. It is argued that the patient is then able to habituate to the trigger and so classically condition to the calm or neutral emotional state that comes once the stress has passed.

Due to the high- intensity exposure in the initial stages the level of fear initially invariably intensifies. It is therefore critical that fear intensities are monitored to ensure the treatment is not stopped until it has subsided again, otherwise the fear will be higher rather than lower post-treatment. In humans this is achieved by grading the fear and not ending exposure until it has at least halved from its starting level. Repeated treatment then aims for complete extinction. There is also said to be a cognitive element in people, suggested to release repressed emotions, and often paired with relaxation techniques during and after exposure. As the treatment can be traumatic human patients also make a clear decision

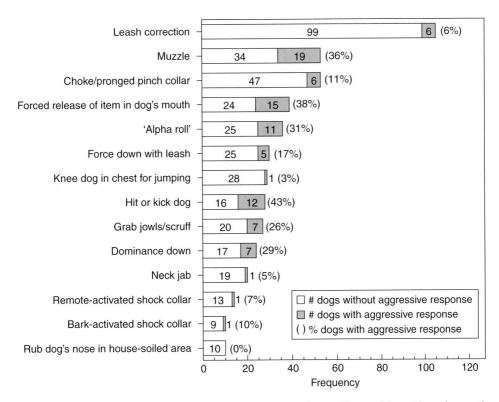

Fig. 56. Percentage of dogs responding aggressively to confrontational or positive-punishment based corrections (Herron *et al.*, 2009. Reproduced with permission from M. Herron).

to 'face their fears' in this way, which is also very likely to impact on its success.

Flooding is used by some practitioners to modify dog behaviour. Because the dog cannot give 'informed consent', exposure is invariably forced. This causes the dog extreme distress, which raises ethical issues regarding its use, places those involved at risk of defensive aggression and is often emotionally stressful for the owner. It also carries significant risk of making the behaviour worse rather than better. Dogs are unable to grade and report their fear levels during treatment. The behaviourist or owner can therefore only rely on the dog's external signs of fear to assess whether it has increased or decreased. This can be unreliable. Although reduction in the signs of fear or stress may be linked to a genuine reduction in fear in some cases, it may also be linked to 'learned helplessness', a state in which the dog gives up fighting the stressor without being any less afraid of it. There is therefore a risk that the treatment may be stopped too soon. If the treatment is stopped whilst the level of fear is higher than the starting point this will lead to an increase in the dog's level of fear and a deterioration in the dog's future behaviour in response to the trigger. If the dog perceives the owner as likely to prevent his escape when exposed to the trigger in the future this may also lead to aggression directed to the owner. Training that involves forcibly exposing a dog to its trigger for fear is therefore not advised.

Environmental Management

Owner behaviour

Many problem behaviours can be addressed by modifying owner behaviour. The first and most important step in doing this is helping the owner understand the reasons for their dog's behaviour. Many owners instinctively change their own behaviour once they understand their dogs. Teaching owners about canine body language is also very effective, both in enabling them to read their dog's body language and understand the effect of their own.

This helps them manage situations better by responding appropriately to the signals their dog is sending.

Teaching clients the effect their own stress or anger may have on their dog, even if it is not directed at him can be beneficial. Making them aware of the importance of behaving consistently to enable the dog to successfully work out ways to behave that increase reward and reduce the likelihood of punishment can also reduce anxiety, frustration and aggression on both sides. Stopping the use of positive punishments that can cause fear, anxiety or be the reason for any aggression will have a further substantial impact on the dog's behaviour. Finally, teaching owners how to use basic training to communicate their wishes to their dog will improve both management and communication.

When suggesting changes to the owner's behaviour it is important to take into account the owner's reasons for having their dog, their own needs and any specific difficulties they may have. The aim is to develop a relationship that is harmonious for both. Focusing too strongly on the dog's needs may increase the chance the owner will choose to rehome or euthanize the dog (discussed below). Equally in some cases the owner's expectations may not be realistic with this – or any – dog. In this case the limitations of the dog's ability to do what is required or for the dog's behaviour to change if they are not willing or able to perform the required training will need to be discussed.

It is commonly recommended that owners change their interactions with their dog in favour of a 'rank reduction' approach to modifying their dog's behaviour. The common methods used are summarized in Tables 12 and 13 (Chapter 4). As discussed in Chapter 4, the theory that underpins these suggestions cannot be scientifically supported and is potentially damaging. Therefore the methods suggested can be either ineffective or, in some cases, harmful. Given the risks, they are best avoided.

Environmental stressors

Identification of environmental stressors is performed in the diagnostic stage. This knowledge can then be used to remove, manage or teach the dog to no longer be worried by them.

Coping strategies

The dog's ability to cope with stressors can be supported by providing an 'escape to safety', perhaps where stressors cannot be removed or whilst desensitization and classical counter-conditioning training is underway. This involves giving the dog a place in which he feels safe and so can retreat to when he feels threatened.

'Escape to safety' is very different to 'escape from danger'. 'Escape from danger' is the dog's attempt to distance himself from a perceived threat. As such the behaviour only occurs once fear has already been triggered. This risks reinforcing the dog's association between the trigger and the unpleasant sensations of fear. It also risks teaching the dog that curiosity or exploratory behaviour may lead to unwanted outcomes and so reduce confidence. Conversely 'escape to safety' is provision of a safe refuge that the dog knows is always there if needed. He can then explore the world safe in the knowledge that a retreat is available. This mimics the behaviour of puppies when they first start to explore outside of the nest and so builds confidence. It also allows the animal to withdraw before reaching the level of fear to avoid this being aggravated.

Key considerations when creating an 'escape to safety' are summarized in Box 7.3 and Fig. 57. If there is no room for a crate or dedicated structure, or the dog does not take to it, household furniture can often be adapted, such as by creating a space under a table or between armchairs.

Desensitization and classical counter-conditioning

The dog's emotional reaction to triggers can be changed through desensitization and counter-conditioning. This will require referral to an accredited behaviourist.

Increased Stimulation

Most dog breeds were created to suit a way of life that has now disappeared. Few dogs still perform the task for which they were intended, and it is increasingly common for all household members to be out for a large part of the day. People do not walk as much as they used to and access to open spaces, especially where dogs can be let off lead, is reducing. People also have higher standards of hygiene than ever before and we live in a risk-adverse society in which guarantees of safety are expected. All of these things adversely affect the typical dog's way of life or acceptance by society, which can result in problem behaviour due to

Box 7.3. Key considerations for an 'escape to safety' den.

- Make sure it is accessible at all times.
- Position away from any stress/fear triggers.
- Enclose on five out of six sides.
- Support with spray or plug-in pheromones.
- Place items the owner has worn or slept with in the den to add a sense of security (depending on the trigger for the animal's fear).
- Line the den with two or more sets of bedding, which are washed in rotation. This balances the reassurance the dog gets from his own scent with hygiene.
- Soundproof with thick blankets or foam wrapped around the outside for noise-phobic dogs. Care should be taken to maintain ventilation and prevent the dog overheating.

- There must be one den per dog where there is conflict between individuals in the house. Care must be taken to ensure there is no competition over access to crates. Referral to an accredited behaviourist will be needed if there is.
- The den must never be used for any kind of punishment and the dog must not be confined in it.
- Some dogs will take a few days to accept their den. It should be set up and left open to allow the dog to habituate to it. The dog should not be pressured to go in but can be encouraged by placing toys or lasting treats inside to classically condition it to positive emotions. The dog could also be fed in the den.

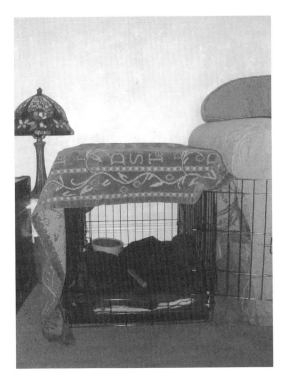

Fig. 57. An example of an 'escape to safety'.

lack of exercise, stimulation and companionship. This type of problem behaviour can be alleviated by improving standards of exercise or stimulation or ensuring a dog's natural drives are fulfilled. There are a number of ways this can be achieved.

Physical exercise

Physical exercise is beneficial for health and weight management. Excess energy may also lead to impulsivity or the dog finding undesirable ways to release it. Ensuring an animal receives sufficient physical exercise is therefore important. However, increasing physical exercise beyond the animal's optimal need has little benefit and may have disadvantages.

There is a current trend for using treadmills or other techniques to force a dog to run for prolonged periods. This type of forced exercise may result in pain or injury due to the dog's inability to control the exercise he undergoes. It also fails to address the cause of the problem behaviour it is intended to prevent. In the short term many dogs will initially be physically tired by the excessive exercise, reducing the performance of all – including unwanted – behaviour. However, as the dog becomes fitter his need for stimulation may actually increase. The reduction in problem behaviour may be prolonged in animals unable to build additional muscle mass, such as those still developing, ageing animals or those that are unwell. However, using this weakness to control behaviour is ethically questionable.

Behavioural stimulation

Physical exercise is not just about health and weight control. It also allows for behavioural stimulation and fulfilment of natural drives such as mock hunting, grooming, territory management and social interaction. These behavioural needs can be fulfilled in ways other than physical exercise where the owner is unable to supply optimal exercise levels. Such methods can also be used to fulfil intellectual needs in intelligent dogs and fulfil drives not addressed by physical exercise.

Feeding

Most animals spend a significant proportion of their time acquiring and consuming food. This fulfils natural drives and generates pleasure associated with these acts for a significant proportion of the day. Modern patterns of feeding dogs have often reduced the amount of time a dog spends eating to a few minutes a day. Therefore increasing the amount of time a dog spends feeding can reduce unwanted behaviour by reducing boredom and fulfilling normal drives. Ways in which this can be achieved are summarized in Table 29.

Sports

There are now a huge number of canine sports to suit almost every different canine pattern of behaviour, owner level of fitness and pocket. The most common of these are summarized in Table 30. Whilst these sports genuinely help direct energy constructively the dog must not be allowed to become so aroused when performing them that it creates rather than controls problem behaviour. The owner's competiveness also should not be allowed to take precedence over the dog's needs and welfare.

Social interaction

Dogs are a social species. They can learn to accept being alone some of the time. How long that is depends on the dog. Young puppies should only be left for a couple of hours at a time, as they not only need regular toilet breaks but also need to be given the opportunity to learn about their environment and how to behave. They are unable to do this is they are alone or confined to a crate for long periods.

Older dogs can cope for longer periods as long as their needs are being met. However, some will still become restless, bored or anxious if left for more than 4 or 5 h. The owner must also be aware that time spent alone at night contributes to the overall time the dog is on his own. Where circumstances necessitate the dog is left for longer than he can cope with, dog walking services or care by others may prevent problem behaviour. Clients should take

Table 29. Activity feeding options.

Method	Description
Active feeding toys	Toys that require the dog to actively engage with them to access the food inside. These can include treat balls, wobblers and puzzle toys. These generally suit treats or dry kibble diets. They are useful for dogs that have energy that needs to be expended.
Passive feeding toys	Toys that contain food that can be removed by chewing or licking. These generally suit wet food. Dry food can be mixed with wet, soaked or soaked and frozen. Liquids can be frozen if the dog is in an area with washable floor coverings. These are useful for dogs that require mental but not physical stimulation. They include Kongs, Busy Buddies and hollow long bones.
Chew toys	Items that require prolonged chewing can occupy a lot of a dog's time, especially for breeds that like to chew. All such items carry a degree of risk, such as splintering in cooked bones, infection with raw bones, teeth fractures if bearing down on Stag Bars or swelling of rawhide chews in the abdomen if large chunks are swallowed. The added calorie intake also has to be considered. However, these drawbacks need to be balanced against the benefits of chewing on welfare and direction of behaviour, and careful supervision can massively reduce risk.
Raw feeding	Raw feeding is controversial and carries certain risks. However, one of its advantages is that it takes much longer for the dog to consume than most processed foods.
Scatter feeding	Dry kibble can be scattered on floors or lawns for the dog to forage.
Training	Using part or even all of the dog's ration as training rewards both occupies their time and their minds. It also increases their responses to training and so control of behaviour.

Table 30. Canine sports.

Sport	Description
Agility	Dogs go over obstacles such as jumps, tunnels and weave poles. Helps control impulsivity and improve owner focus.
Flyball	Dogs go over jumps, release a ball from a box and then return in a four-dog relay. It provides an outlet for chase behaviour, but little impulse control.
Tracking, trailing and scent work	The dog is taught to follow a trail on the ground or in the air, or to find hidden objects either outdoors or in the house.
Schutzhund, working trials and protection sports	Involves tracking, obedience and protection work. The latter variously requires controlled apprehension, attack and release of a stooge 'offender'.
Sled racing	Teams of dogs pull a sledge. Competition involves timed races.
Rally O	Dog and handler perform obedience training around a course.
Earth and field trials	Competitions testing dog's working ability, e.g. retrieving, pointing and flushing.
Musical canine freestyle	Dog and owner perform obedience training, tricks and dance to music.
Obedience	The dog and handler perform and are judged on a series of obedience commands according to set criteria.

great care when choosing a dog walker or day-care provider as the industry is currently unregulated. Time spent alone at night can also be reduced by using a baby gate rather than a solid door to exclude the dog from the bedroom where owners do not want the dog in the room with them.

Owners should ensure they make time each day to interact actively with their dog. This can be through games, training, affection or massage. They should ensure interactions are positive and wanted by the dog. The dog's desire to be petted can be tested by stroking briefly then stopping whilst keeping the hand close by. A dog that is enjoying the interaction will seek further fuss.

It is also important to ensure the dog has sufficient interaction with other dogs, especially during the early months and years. Puppies need to develop social skills with other puppies and adult dogs. This is discussed more in Chapters 10 and 11. Adult free play is also emotionally and behaviourally beneficial. It provides a suitable outlet to expend energy and keeps the dog's social skills honed.

There are certain rules of etiquette to be observed when allowing dogs to play. Not all dogs are sociable so owners should control their dog's approach of other dogs. If the other dog is being kept on lead etiquette dictates the owner does not allow their own dog to approach it. They should instead recall their dog and either put him back on lead or keep him under close control depending on his reliability until they can ask the other owner if it is safe for their dog to approach. There are now a number of campaigns that indicate where a dog is on lead because he does not enjoy the approach of other

dogs or strangers, rather than some other reason such as poor recall. Yellow Dog UK (see Appendix 1) and Space Dogs (USA) use a yellow ribbon attached to the dogs lead to signal that a dog needs space. They also sell dog coats and bandanas, owner T shirts, vests and caps, lead covers and neck ties. DINOS (Dogs In Need Of Space) provides similar products and posters. Dogs that are off lead are usually friendly but there is always the risk they are not, perhaps because the person walking them is unaware of their behaviour or is simply irresponsible. Some dogs may not be aggressive but may be intolerant of boisterous or rude dogs or may be possessive of dogs approaching their owner or trying to take their ball. It is therefore beneficial to teach dogs to always return to their owner from a young age before they are allowed to play and intermittently during play so interactions can be managed.

Diet

The potential effect of diet on behaviour was discussed in Chapter 2. The presiding veterinary surgeon needs to be consulted before any change is made to the dog's diet to modify behaviour so they may consider physiological or medical needs.

Moving the dog on to a diet suitable for his age, size and activity level can help where the existing diet is inappropriate. Trial periods on a quality complete dog food can indicate whether poor-quality diet, specific ingredients or artificial colours are having an adverse impact on the dog's behaviour. Blood sugar fluctuations can be corrected by providing smaller more frequent meals, avoiding diets high in sugar and ensuring the animal's diet has a significant proportion of slow burn carbohydrates.

Protein/carbohydrate balance

The effects of an imbalance between protein and carbohydrate were discussed in Chapter 2. Modifying diet can help correct this and increase serotonin levels in the brain, reducing anxiety and aggression. This is achieved by feeding increased carbohydrate levels to trigger insulin release, which in turn increases uptake of large neutral amino acids (LNAA) into muscle. This increases the ratio of tryptophan:LNAA and so the proportion of tryptophan hydroxylase crossing the blood–brain barrier and so serotonin levels in the brain. Serotonin production may further be facilitated by ensuring optimal vitamin B6 (pyridoxine) levels, due to its activity in serotonin production.

Docosahexaenoic acid

Docosahexaenoic acid (DHA) is an omega 3 fatty acid found in fish, eggs and some meat. It plays a significant role in brain and retina development. A lack of DHA has been linked to dementia. Some puppy diets contain supplementation with DHA as it is suggested to make puppies easier to train. However, studies performed so far have been based on comparing elevated and deficient dietary DHA. To be of value studies are needed comparing elevated to recommended daily allowances of DHA.

Neutering

Neutering of animals may be performed prophylactically or for the treatment of various medical conditions. It is also often recommended for behavioural management. However, its effects may not be as predictable or far reaching as was historically suggested.

Castration

Castration removes the testicles and so the principal site for production of testosterone and, to a lesser extent, oestrogen. Castration therefore reduces, but does not totally eliminate, testosterone from the circulation. The effects of testosterone on behaviour are summarized in Table 31.

The precise effect of the removal of testosterone will depend on the developmental stage at which castration is performed. Increased levels of testosterone in the foetus increases receptor sensitivity to it, increasing male patterns of behaviour when testosterone levels rise at puberty. Pre-parturient testosterone also affects organization of neurons for male patterns of behaviour, which will still occur regardless of whether the dog produces testosterone after birth. As such, some male behaviour occurs even where castration is performed before puberty. Where castration is performed post-puberty further patterns of male behaviour are also likely to have developed, both due to neural organization and learning. Castration can also impact on some physiological conditions, which in turn influence behaviour, e.g. hypothyroidism. A summary of research so far into the effects of castration is given in Table 32.

Given the wide variation in the potential effect of castration its usefulness as a method of changing problem behaviour needs to be assessed on a case by case basis, once the cause for the problem behaviour has been determined and the dog's overall behaviour understood. This is best performed

Table 31. The behavioural effects of testosterone.

Effect	Discussion
Sexual competition	Increased competitive aggression linked to reproduction, especially in the presence of reproductive triggers, e.g. a female in oestrus.
Attention	Increased focus on a stimulus and reduced ease of distraction from it.
Risk taking	Increased risk taking and impulsivity.
Intensity of aggression	Increased use of threat and increased intensity, speed and duration of aggressive incidents.
Strength	Physical androgenization may increase power and strength.
Confidence	Testosterone is higher in confident and successful individuals, increasing their willingness to use threat on subsequent occasions, although the direction of influence is unclear.
Reduced fear	Testosterone reduces fearful responses (van Honk *et al.*, 2005).

Table 32. The behavioural effects of castration.

Effect	Discussion
Fertility and mating behaviour	Testosterone levels drop rapidly but the dog is still fertile for up to 6 weeks and many continue to mate for many months post-castration.
Roaming	Castration normally leads to a rapid and consistent reduction in roaming.
Mounting	May reduce when linked to mating or masturbation but not if due to other triggers
Scent marking	Scenting associated with mating behaviour is reduced but territorial marking is not.
Aggression – sexual	Fighting between entire males for a mate is generally reduced. This may be the cause for sporadic fighting between entire males even though the owner is unaware of a bitch in heat in the vicinity.
Aggression – other	The speed, intensity and duration of aggressive interactions, and the dog's confidence to challenge may be reduced following castration. However, removal of the confidence and fear inhibition effects of testosterone may make fearful aggression worse. Testosterone is known to potentiate exogenous serotonin, so its removal may also reduce the latter's calming and sociability effects, increasing aggressive responses.

by an accredited behaviourist in liaisan with the veterinary surgeon.

Circulating testosterone reduces after 24 h. A small amount will continue to be produced by the adrenals throughout the animal's life, however this is thought to have minimal effect on behaviour.

In many cases castration will need to be supported by a behaviour modification programme to remove learnt patterns of behaviour, address underpinning drives (where not sexual) or to prevent castration being replaced by a different unwanted behaviour, e.g. in dogs that used to roam but now stay at home.

Cryptorchid

Unilateral or bilateral cryptorchidism may affect testosterone levels. The retained testicle(s) will not produce normal sperm but will continue to produce testosterone, albeit at a lower level. If the animal is bilaterally cryptorchid he is therefore less likely to show behaviours associated with testosterone. In humans, retained testicles produce increased levels of testosterone during puberty. Retained testicles are also more likely to become neoplastic, potentially resulting in increased testosterone levels

Ovariohysterectomy

As reproductive hormones in the female are cyclic it is somewhat easier to predict the effects of ovariohysterectomy. The behavioural effects of the relevant hormones are summarized in Table 4.

Where unwanted behaviour occurs in cycles linked to reproductive hormones and completely regresses once the cycle has passed, neutering is likely to resolve the problem. For example, aggressive behaviour clearly linked to the period of prolactin production, even where no other overt clinical signs of false pregnancy are seen, should not recur post-neutering. Equally, bitches that only fight as one or both of their seasons approach should also fall back into the status quo once hormones are removed from the scenario. However, it must be borne in mind that only those hormones produced by the Graafian follicle, corpus luteum or placenta are removed. Pituitary hormones such as follicle stimulating hormone (FSH) and luteinizing hormone (LH) are known to increase post-spay.

If the behaviour does not follow the pattern of reproductive hormones then neutering is unlikely to be beneficial. There is some evidence to suggest aggressive bitches neutered under 12 months of age may be made worse by early neutering.

Pharmacology

Some behaviour problems may respond to medication. Use of medication is intended to facilitate not replace behaviour modification. The principal reasons for using medication in behaviour management or modification are summarized in Table 33.

As medication does not remedy the problem it is important that a behaviour modification programme is implemented concurrent to or after use of medication, depending on its purpose or effect. It is generally useful for the behaviourist accepting

Table 33. Reasons for using pharmaceuticals in behaviour cases.

Reason	Description
Short-term management	For transient problems, e.g. firework phobias. They may also be justified as a short-term first aid measure where the behaviour poses an immediate risk to the animal or others, compromises the animal's quality of life or where time or owner pressure risks the animal being euthanized.
Re-establishing emotional homeostasis	Following disruption due to chronic stress or anxiety.
Adjusting the animal's emotional state	Artificially adjusting the animal's emotional state can facilitate behaviour modification, especially in long-standing behaviours that have become entrenched or where behavioural triggers cannot be avoided or sufficiently controlled. Drugs having this effect may also be used in cases of severe compulsions to prevent them becoming a habit whilst behaviour modification is underway.

the case to see the dog before medication is started so they can assess behaviour before the medication takes effect.

Prescription drugs

Tri-cyclic antidepressants

Tri-cyclic antidepressants (TCAs) increase circulating levels of serotonin and noradrenaline by inhibiting re-uptake at the synaptic cleft and antagonizing adrenergic neurotransmitters. Over time they also increase the number of serotonin and noradrenaline receptors at the nerve endings, increasing the efficiency of neurotransmitter-receptor binding. The effect of TCAs is to elevate mood due to increased serotonin and to reduce anxiety and panic due to reduced adrenergic effects. Examples include clomipramine, imipramine and amitriptyline.

Selected serotonin re-uptake inhibitors

Selected serotonin re-uptake inhibitors (SSRIs) inhibit re-uptake and increase the number of receptors for serotonin only. Due to their specificity they are up to three times more effective at increasing levels of active serotonin than TCAs. They also have lower side effects. An example is fluoxetine.

Mono-amine oxidase inhibitors

Mono-amine oxidase A (MAO-A) is responsible for the re-uptake of serotonin, adrenaline and noradrenaline in the dog. MAO-B is responsible for re-uptake of histamine and dopamine. Both act on re-uptake of phenethylamine, which is a releasing agent for noradrenaline and dopamine. Mono-amine oxidase inhibitors (MAOIs) inhibit MAO and so increase synaptic levels of these neurotransmitters, depending on which MAO they affect. An example of a drug active on MAO-B is selegeline.

Benzodiazepines

Benzodiazepines potentiate the binding of GABA, the principal inhibitory neurotransmitter, in the limbic system. The effect is to reduce excitation and anxiety. They may also increase social interaction and have mild retrograde amnesic qualities, which are effective up to 1 h before and for the duration of the treatment.

Disinhibition caused by benzodiazepines may cause increased aggression and occasional paradoxical hyper-excitation. There is also an inhibition of learning due to effects on NMDA/glutamate receptor. They are therefore only suitable for short-term management of behaviour and cannot be used to support a behaviour modification programme. Examples include alprazolam and diazepam.

Beta-antagonists

Beta-antagonists block the effects of adrenaline and noradrenaline. As a result they inhibit fight or flight effects. They also reduce melatonin binding, so may interfere with sleep patterns, and act as a serotonin receptor agonist. An example is propranolol.

Acepromazine

Acepromazine is an alpha-adrenergic and dopamine antagonist. It inhibits vasoconstriction, gluconeogenesis and stimulation of arousal centres. It also inhibits reward systems. At moderate doses the dog becomes unresponsive to stimulation with lowered arousal and behavioural responses. However, he will also become lethargic with slowed reactions and blunted decision making. This may lead to irritability and poor decision making, resulting in increased aggression. Long-term use of acepromazine in cows causes chronic stress and has also been suggested to increase sensitivity to noise.

Nutraceuticals and herbal preparations

Valerian

Valerian is a herbal product found to act on melatonin receptors. It therefore increases sleepiness. It also has a possible effect on GABA receptors. Clinical trials show it helps induce onset of sleep and may reduce anxiety or aggression. However, production does not enjoy the controls offered by pharmaceutical products and so the chemical composition of plants grown for its production may vary with environment, time of year and regional genetic variations. Different preparation techniques may also affect the final product.

Alpha-casozepine

Alpha-casozepine is a nutraceutical derived from alpha S1 (αS1) casein in milk. This is recognized to have calming qualities due to its affinity for GABA receptors. The effects of αS1 are greater in neo-

nates as their digestive system favours trypsin over pepsin, which is more efficient at digesting milk. The presentation in pharmacologically prepared alpha-casozepine facilitates adult digestion.

Tests on normal rats and humans showed reductions in stress within 24 h. Studies of cats and dogs with established anxiety disorders showed gradual improvement over a 56 day period. Effects in the first 14 days were low.

Pheromones

The role and behavioural effects of naturally occurring pheromones was introduced in Chapter 5. This effect can also be manipulated through use of synthetic analogues. In the case of the dog the only pheromone to be synthetically recreated is the appeasing pheromone (appeasine) produced in the ears and the mammary sulcus of the lactating bitch to reassure her offspring.

The claimed effects include reduction or prevention of fear or anxiety-related signs, increased sense of familiarity and security and acceleration of desensitization and counter-conditioning due to increased sense of familiarity. They are suggested to act synergistically with benzodiazepines.

Presentations

The pheromone is available in a number of presentations, each suited to a different use. These are outlined in Table 34.

Table 34. Presentations for synthetic dog-appeasing pheromones.

Presentation	Discussion
Pump spray	Primarily suited to transient situations such as car travel, visits to the vets or when introducing a dog to a specific location, e.g. a new crate or kennel. It can be applied directly to surfaces or to a bandana placed around the dog's neck. The pheromone is carried in an alcohol base, which must be allowed to evaporate before the dog is exposed to it. Each application lasts 2–3 h.
Diffuser	The pheromone is suspended in a carrier base, which is heated and diffused through a unit plugged into a standard electrical socket. It is suited to generalized fear/anxiety that only occurs in the home, e.g. house visitors, anxiety-based separation-related problems and firework phobias. It can also be used to establish a puppy or dog in a new environment, e.g. hospital stay, rescue sanctuary. Time needs to be given to allow the pheromone concentration to reach the required saturation after being plugged in. The unit needs to be left on all the time so this is maintained.
Collar	The pheromone is impregnated into a plastic collar. It is recommended for generalized fear or anxiety that occurs outside or both inside and outside the home, e.g. fear of strangers, noise sensitivity, traffic, other dogs etc. The collar needs to be in gentle contact with the skin so body heat warms and releases the pheromone. The effect is normally achieved rapidly and lasts for about 4 weeks.

Contraindications

There have been occasional anecdotal reports of adverse behavioural reactions such as avoidance and hyper-excitation where a collar is used. The collar should not be used on sore or broken skin. The pheromone only affects the behaviour of dogs.

Occasionally use of pheromones may increase aggression due to reduction in the inhibition of fearful or withdrawal behaviour. Use on one dog in a multi-dog household may also disrupt relationships. It may increase confidence in a dog more prone to flight than fight or may make any dogs not wearing the collar excessively curious towards those that are. Care must therefore be taken if there is any conflict between dogs living together. Use in situations where unavoidably stressful handling or treatment will be performed may also create mixed signals. For example, spray used in a hospital kennel combined with invasive treatment performed in the kennel may confuse the dog about whether it is a safe place or not.

Alternative Therapies

The alternative therapies discussed here remain controversial. However, it is important to be aware of the current evidence linked to them to enable objective discussion with clients regarding their use and efficacy.

Aromatherapy

Aromatherapy uses plant extracts for the treatment of a range of medical conditions. In animals the extracts are normally inhaled. The plants used are often similar to those used in herbal medicine but are obtained by distillation and therefore are highly concentrated. As aromatherapy is a recognized treatment it can only be given under the direction of a veterinary surgeon other when an owner is treating their own pet.

Use of lavender oil has been shown to have a positive effect on dogs although it is not clear if this is due to aromatherapy or distraction. Smell triggers the limbic system, which links emotion to memory. It is therefore suggested that any aroma used to manage behaviour in dogs must already have a classically conditioned link between the smell and a positive emotion to be effective. It must be borne in mind that strong aromas may affect normal pheromonal or other olfactory signalling.

Bach flowers

Bach flowers are claimed to treat emotional states linked to illness. Some owners may therefore try using them to help a dog showing emotional distress such as fear or anxiety. Rescue Remedy is a particularly common Bach flower combination in general use both in humans and animals. Studies have shown that Bach flowers can have a strong placebo effect on the behaviour of people when used to treat their own symptoms. If the owner's expectation of efficacy extends to the treatment of their dog, any 'placebo effect' may not only impact on their perception of their dog's behaviour, but any related changes in the owner's behaviour may in turn have a real impact on the behaviour of the dog.

Tellington Touch

Tellington Touch body work, or TTouch, involves using a range of light circular hand movements to stimulate the skin. The animal's response to touches is initially evaluated to enable suitable touches to be selected. Each touch is performed in a specialized way according to the intended effect. Practitioners undergo an extensive course of training.

Massage is known to trigger positive neural responses and production of endogenous opioids. Stroking also stimulates oxytocin production, which may elevate mood and slow the heart. However, to be beneficial it needs to be performed in a way the dog and owner find mutually beneficial.

The research supporting the efficacy of TTouch only considers the effects of a course of treatment without comparison to other forms of massage (Bernhard *et al.*, 2009). There is therefore nothing to suggest it is superior. However, following the methods recommended does ensure the owner delivers massage in a way the dog should find pleasurable and teaches them to observe and accommodate their dog's responses to it. This should help maximize its beneficial effects.

Face and body wraps

Body pressure wraps such as the Anxiety Wrap® and Thundershirt are suggested to calm behaviour through deep pressure. It is widely recognized that touch is pleasurable, especially deep touch such as hugging, through the release of endorphins. The principle that pressure from an inanimate object such as a wrap or 'hug machine' may also be beneficial has also been proposed and supported for at least some participants (Grandin, 1992). However, studies so far into use of pressure wraps for autistic children have not found any suggestion they calm or reduce stereotypic behaviour, and in at least one case were found to make behaviour worse (Reichow *et al.*, 2009; Stephenson and Carter, 2009; Hodgetts, 2010; Hodgetts *et al.*, 2011).

Current research on body wraps in dogs is limited. Cottam *et al.* (2013) found 89% of owners reported a body wrap to be at least partially effective at reducing their dog's signs of anxiety during thunder storms after five uses. The effect gradually increased with successive use. As the study sample was small, relied on owner report and did not employ a placebo the results must be interpreted with caution. The study also recognized that the reduction seen in most of the signs measured would occur equally whether the wrap reduces anxiety or inhibits activity due to an increase in anxiety. The notable exception to this was the reduction in shaking, suggesting a genuine reduction in anxiety not just in locomotion. However, a further study incorporating measurement of physiological values would make this more reliable.

Face wraps are available with the intention of reducing barking. The increased effort required to do so when the wrap is in place may make it effective. However, it does not change the dog's motivation for barking. They therefore risk creating frustration, anxiety or redirection of problem behaviour elsewhere.

Rehoming and Euthanasia

Canine behaviour, with all its complex influences and its inextricable association with human needs and behaviour cannot always be corrected. Genetically driven behaviours or those hard-wired early in development may need lifelong management rather than correction, which not all owners are able or willing to give. Changes in circumstances such as illness, disability or relationship breakdown may mean an owner is no longer able to provide for a dog's behavioural needs. The presence or birth of children can impact on an owner's willingness to tolerate certain behaviours or their ability to safely manage and address some problems. It is frustratingly common for people to acquire dogs that are highly unsuitable for them, such as working dogs for a pet home or dogs that require much more exercise and stimulation than the owner is willing or able to give. Some owners simply do not have

the time, skills, resources or inclination to rehabilitate their dog. Even where they do, if the emotional bond has irretrievably broken down they may not have the heart to. Relinquishment of the dog then becomes the only option the owners have or are prepared to consider.

Rehoming

When a client approaches a veterinary and behavioural professional to discuss relinquishment they must provide impartial and realistic advice. Rehoming is preferred where possible. However, there are a number of considerations to be taken into account when deciding if this is appropriate.

Suitability of the dog

Before rehoming, the dog's prognosis for improvement has to be evaluated. Some problems have genetic drives or arise due to strong behaviour patterns established during the developmental period. The animal's ability to cope with novelty or stress or to respond to training can also have congenital or physiological causes that cannot be changed with behaviour modification. These dogs will require lifelong management. All dogs find rehoming considerably more distressing than is perhaps recognized and some may not cope, especially old or dispositionally anxious dogs.

Suitability of new owners

If the dog's behaviour is problematic in his current home this immediately makes rehoming more challenging. It is essential the prospective new owner is fully aware of the problem behaviour and is willing to commit to addressing it. They also need to be objectively assessed to ensure they are genuinely able to do so. Sentimentality or a failure to accept the reality of the problem behaviour will often lead prospective owners to adopt a dog they are unable realistically to help. This invariably leads to repeated relinquishment, which generally leads to a further deterioration in behaviour.

Life in kennels versus euthanasia

The reality of dog behaviour is that not every problem dog can be rehomed. Even where a dog has every possibility of full rehabilitation a home may not be able to be found, or it may be decided the risk to the welfare of humans or other animals during rehabilitation is too great for it to be allowed.

Whether such dogs should live their life out in a rescue establishment is a matter of personal ethics. Euthanasia can be defined as 'painless killing to relieve suffering' (RCVS, 2012). This applies equally to emotional suffering as it does to physical. Euthanizing a dog on behavioural grounds is a decision no-one wants to take or takes lightly. However, there are welfare considerations to life-long incarceration. Therefore the dog's ability to cope with kennel life must be assessed and each case decided on its own merits. Where the animal's five freedoms can be fulfilled and he is able to lead a dignified and enjoyable life, long-term kennelling may be acceptable. However, if confining a dog to kennels for a lifetime causes emotional distress that cannot be ameliorated with environmental management, enrichment or even medication then their quality of life has to be questioned. In this situation it takes a stronger and more caring professional to alleviate the dog from its current and future suffering. Pretending that euthanasia never has to or should happen is avoiding facing and dealing with the reality of some behaviours and the welfare implications for all involved.

PART 2
Handling in Practice

Introduction

Management of potentially aggressive dogs is a key part of the veterinary nurse or technician's everyday role. Historically, training in how to handle dogs in the practice focused on various methods of restraint to keep the dog still and prevent injury to staff. However, our knowledge of canine behaviour has grown enormously in recent years. We are therefore now able to use that behavioural understanding to reduce the dog's perceived need to use threat, reducing the need for physical restraint in many situations. This carries many benefits.

Staff productivity and morale

Physical control of dogs is time consuming and often involves multiple staff members. Reduced aggressive incidents can therefore improve productivity. A reduction in incidents also improves staff morale, enabling them to focus on providing the support and care they no doubt envisaged when they chose the profession.

Patient welfare

Taking steps to reduce a dog's perception that he needs to use aggression will improve his welfare. As discussed in Chapter 5, a dog that is showing affective (i.e. non-predatory) aggression is in distress. The trigger for this can vary, but in the practice it is almost invariably due to feeling his safety is under threat. The aggression being shown is therefore intended to make staff withdraw however fearless, confident or intimidating the dog may seem. Avoiding that situation arising protects the dog from such distress and so protects his welfare. It also reduces the chance he will learn to be fearful of the practice and so use a higher level of aggression in future visits.

Client satisfaction

Clients often judge a practice by how their dog behaves and is handled. If they feel their dog is happy at the practice and do not have to observe him being forcibly restrained their experience is far more likely to be a positive one, which will bond them to the practice.

Time investment

As such, although the measures discussed in the following chapters do require changes in approach and some time investment, this is easily compensated for by reductions in time needed to physically control dogs that have become difficult to handle, staff and patient welfare, and client loyalty.

Trigger Stacking in Practice

Although preventing all aggression in practice is unrealistic, the risk it will occur can be lowered by applying the 'trigger stacking' model discussed in Chapter 5. Table 35 discusses the factors that will either push a dog closer to or reduce a dog's aggression threshold in the practice.

The potential for these triggers to combine and cause a dog to use aggression is depicted in Fig. 58.

Preventing aggression

The approach to preventing aggression in practice used here aims to identify the factors influencing each dog's use of aggression and taking steps to reduce those that can be controlled this prevents them stacking together to push the dog over his threshold. The steps may be taken at the time of, before or after the visit. How to do this is discussed in Chapters 8 and 9.

Table 35. Factors that may push a dog closer to or reduce his aggression threshold in the veterinary practice.

Factor	Discussion
Being in pain or feeling ill	Causes the dog to defend the painful part and increases irritability.
Unfamiliar place or smells	Some dogs find anything new or unfamiliar unsettling.
Owner stress	Dogs pick up on owner behaviour and mood, especially stress. An owner's worry about their dog's health or behaviour in the practice may increase the risk of aggressive behaviour.
Other dog's stress pheromones or behaviour	The behaviour of other dogs and stress pheromones emitted by other current or past patients may act as a signal of threat, increasing the likelihood of aggression. Pheromones can last in the atmosphere for some time due to protection from binding proteins.
Restraint and manipulation	The choice between 'fight' and 'flight' is affected by the dog's perception of his options. Firm restraint or manipulation may result in the dog feeling his 'flight' option is compromised, increasing the likelihood he will use 'fight'.
Invasive procedures	Genuinely painful procedures may understandably increase defensive behaviour. Many dogs also become concerned at non-painful procedures such as temperature taking, claw clipping and examination.
Human approach or behaviour	Human approach, such as standing over, staring at or reaching for the dog may inadvertently mimic dog threat postures (see Chapter 4). Cornering, corrections, alpha rolling or actual or perceived anger will also escalate fear and use of aggression.
Past experiences	A visit to the practice typically involves either illness, injury or invasive prophylactic treatment. Dogs can quickly start to associate being there with pain or fear, reducing the aggression threshold.
Dog's pre-existing triggers	Stimuli that already worry the dog and naturally occur in the practice will increase fear and so push the dog closer to his aggression threshold. This may include things like noise, strangers or other dogs.
Temperament of the dog	Factors such as genes, early experiences, past experience outside of the practice, use of excessive punishment or the dog's relationship with their owner may affect use of aggression.

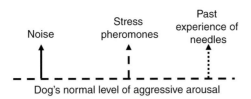

Level at which dog will show aggression

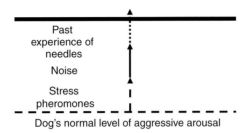

Level at which dog will show aggression

Reduced level at which dog shows
aggression due to pain or illness

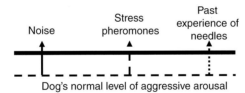

Fig. 58. Trigger stacking in the veterinary practice.

8 Managing the Environment

Managing the practice environment can help reduce the risk that a dog may become distressed or fearful, and so the likelihood he will use aggression when approached or handled. Ways in which this can be achieved are summarized below.

The Waiting Room

The waiting room not only creates a first impression for the practice but also influences the emotional state of the dog when he enters the consultation room. If a dog or his owner have become anxious whilst waiting the dog is already on the upward spiral to an aggressive outburst. Taking steps to help keep the dog calm from the moment they enter the practice door will therefore go a long way towards preventing aggression both in the waiting room and for the rest of the visit.

Design

Unless at the design stage, changing waiting room layout may not be practical. However, there are various gold-standard design features that can be borne in mind if there is some flexibility in layout or if structural modifications are being considered.

One way entry and exit

Dogs avoid direct face to face contact on initial greeting. A single entry and exit point forces dogs to meet face to face if one leaves as another arrives. Installation of a separate exit prevents this from occurring. Where this is not practical full-length safety glass doors avoid clients and dogs being taken by surprise. Suitably worded signs and a dedicated space for retreat can encourage a client to step aside when they see another dog coming through the door, even if their dog has no issues.

Reception desk away from entrance

Clients invariably need to spend time at the reception desk with their dog both on arrival and before departure. Siting this away from the entry and exit prevents face to face meetings or the congregation of dogs in a confined space. Where this is not possible, active management of queues by providing a waiting area away from the door can help reduce the number of dogs at reception at one time. Full-length glass doors and suitably worded signs can also help, as above.

Cubicles

Dogs that are fearful of or aggressive to other dogs can become highly stressed if expected to sit in the same room as another dog for any period of time. Dogs that are fearful for other reasons also typically like to retreat to a place they see as safe. Ideal waiting room design comprises seating arranged in cubicles. Screens or racking can also be used to create the same effect where space allows (see Figs 59 to 61).

Separate dog and cat areas

Separate waiting areas for dogs and cats are often advocated to reduce stress for the cat. However, this can be equally beneficial in reducing dog aggression by preventing excitation, which can lower self-control in a trigger situation.

Air circulation

When dogs are distressed they release pheromones signalling this to others. These stay in the environment for prolonged periods after the dog emitting them has gone, which can have an effect on every dog that enters the waiting room afterwards. Ensuring good ventilation and rapid air changes can help reduce this effect. The use of the appeasing

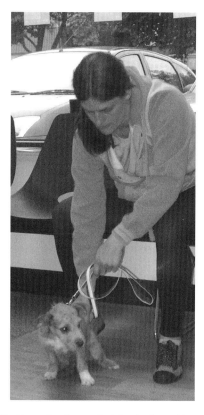

Fig. 59. Example of a worried dog in the waiting room.

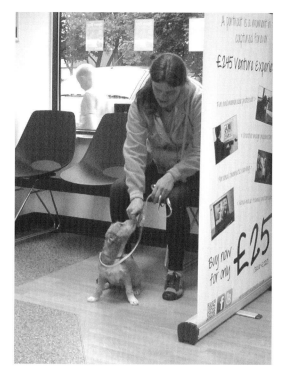

Fig. 60. Use of a screen and lures to help the dog feel more relaxed.

pheromone Adaptil™ can also help reduce the impact of any negative pheromones left behind (see below).

Pheromones

The use of synthetic pheromones in dog behaviour was introduced in Chapter 7. A study of the specific relevance of using Adaptil™ in the waiting and consulting rooms was performed by Mills *et al.* (2006). The study showed significant reductions in anxiety and increases in relaxation when a diffuser was installed. This did not translate to a reduction in actual aggression shown on examination in the study. However, the reductions in anxiety and improvements in relaxation would help reduce the likelihood of aggression when combined with other measures. They would also reduce development of negative associations to the practice that may trigger aggression on subsequent visits through learning. As such, use of a diffuser in the waiting room can be beneficial.

Where this is not possible clients with fearful and easily distressed dogs could be advised to use Adaptil™ spray on a bandanna around the dog's neck. The spray should be applied to the bandanna and left in another room for 10 min to allow the alcohol the pheromone is carried in to evaporate. The bandana should be applied before leaving home to maximize its calming effect and minimize stress build-up during the journey.

Whilst the usual effect of Adaptil™ is to reduce anxiety, occasionally it may make aggression more likely due to increased confidence. This is not common in fear-based aggression and so should not preclude its use in fearful dogs. However, the owner and practice should both bear this in mind, even in dogs that have not previously shown aggression.

Comfort

Many dogs, especially those that are old or arthritic, find walking on slippery floors painful or distressing. Provision of non-slip mats can help reduce such distress or prevent pain that may add to the animal's

Chapter 8

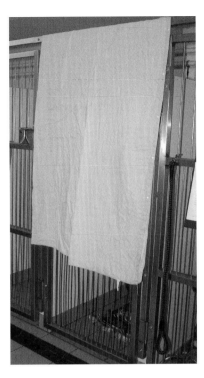

Fig. 61. Covering the top half of a full-height kennel can prevent looking down on a dog and so the potential to appear threatening.

irritability. Some dogs also find sitting or lying on cold hard floors unpleasant, adding to their pain, irritability or distress. Provision of soft bedding may help prevent this. This can be provided by the practice, or clients can be encouraged to bring bedding in with them. Worried dogs may prefer this due to the added reassurance bedding with their own familiar smell gives. It is important the owner understands that the greatest benefit is derived if the bedding has been used for at least a few days prior to the visit. Whilst they may prefer to bring freshly laundered bedding into a public place, it is the smell that comes with use that offers the sense of security and so reduction in fear or stress to the dog.

Managing waiting room behaviour

Reception is a busy place and staff are often distracted from clients waiting for their appointment. However, keeping one eye on the behaviour of both dog and client can prevent escalation of problem situations.

It is best for all concerned if dogs that do not settle well in the waiting room wait outside, in the car (weather permitting) or in a spare consulting room. This principle should apply equally to noisy and boisterous dogs as it does to fearful or aggressive ones. Doing so not only prevents the affected dog's arousal level rising prior to the consultation, but also lessens the impact on the stress levels of the owner and other visitors to the practice. Tact is needed when making this suggestion so the client is not made to feel embarrassed or that they are an inconvenience. By asking the client if they would feel more comfortable in a consulting room/the car park/their car it suggests this is being recommended for their and their dog's benefit rather than because they have caused a problem for anyone else. A practice protocol for informing the staff member conducting consultations where the patient is will need to be developed to prevent confusion.

Reception staff can also help prevent dogs being pushed closer to their aggression threshold if they monitor the behaviour of apparently calm dogs. This can change suddenly and owners may not be aware of early signs that there is conflict brewing between the dogs or their dog is worried. Any signs of low-level stress or worry should be intercepted before the situation escalates (see Fig. 21). If the problem is arising between two dogs the clients should be asked to prevent their dogs approaching each other or be asked to turn their dogs so they cannot look at each other. If this is not sufficient it may be useful for one of the clients to move to another part of the room or to wait elsewhere, as above.

Weighing

Many dogs find being walked on to scales stressful. Cover scales with non-slip mats or a towel to make them more inviting, stand on the scale as the dog steps on to prevent it rocking or choose scales flush with the floor. Ensure the scale has plenty of space at both ends so the dog can be walked on without feeling he is being cornered. Use treats to lure and reward dogs for stepping on where not contraindicated. It may also be beneficial to weigh the dog immediately after arrival to allow time for him to relax again before being taken into the consultation room.

The Consultation or Examination Room

The consultation or examination room needs to be of adequate size and to be uncluttered to prevent the dog feeling trapped or claustrophobic. Ambient temperature should be maintained so as to avoid hyper- or hypothermia. Design should exclude external noise.

Ideally dogs should be examined away from other animals and staff not immediately involved in the procedure. This is usual for examinations during consultations. However, where the dog is taken away from the client for examination or is being examined whilst in hospital it is common for this to take place in a busy communal 'prep' or treatment room. In many cases this will house multiple examination tables being used by other staff and animals, or may be a thoroughfare. The activity, noise or presence of other people or animals may increase arousal (both fearful and excitement) in some dogs, reducing their threshold for aggression. This can be avoided by utilizing unused consulting rooms, non-sterile procedure rooms (e.g. X-ray, grooming or dental) or even a corner of the stock room at the first signs that a dog is excited or worried.

Routine cleaning of surfaces and management of air circulation will help remove stress pheromones between patients.

The Hospital

Dogs that are hospitalized will invariably have elevated stress levels. This interferes with both management and recovery. Managing the hospital environment can help minimize the impact of this.

Allocation and management of the kennel

Each kennel can be graded according to the level of stress it is likely to generate. Factors to consider are summarized in Table 36. Dogs can then be matched to the most suitable kennel according to their need for companionship or peace. Cover the top half of full-height kennel doors to avoid people passing looking down on the dog, which may increase stress (see Fig. 61). They can get down to the dog's levels to greet if needed. Half of the bottom of the cage door can also be covered to give the dog a place to hide if required. Avoid completely covering the dog's view out of the kennel if possible as dogs tend to be more worried if they are unable to see out at all and so monitor for the approach of a 'threat'.

Control of visual contact

Some dogs are comforted by the visual presence of others. However, others may become fearful or

Table 36. Factors to consider when assessing the stress factor of a kennel.

Factor	Discussion
Passing traffic	How many people will walk past the kennel during the day and will they have other dogs with them?
Noise levels	How close is the kennel to sources of noise both from within the practice and outside?
Handling required	Higher kennels require the dog to be handled to get him in and out.
Lighting	Is artificial lighting needed, which may be more stressful that natural light?
Overlooking other dogs	Does the kennel overlook other dogs?

excited, neither of which is desirable. The behavioural history and observation of initial visual contact of other dogs will help establish each dog's tendency. This can then be managed as necessary. The use of screens to prevent eye contact is preferable where kennel design does not do so, as it allows the dog to still see out of his kennels whilst restricting sight of other dogs. If this is not practical, blankets can be used to cover three-quarters of the kennel door as above.

Avoidance of invasive procedures in the kennel

If a dog is difficult to handle it is tempting to perform any medical interventions needed in the kennel rather than trying to get him out. However, this raises anxiety by forming associations between being in the kennel and things the animal undoubtedly finds unpleasant, even if they do not show it. It is therefore best to remove the animal for all procedures whenever possible.

Incorporation of positive interactions into the treatment plan

If staff only interact with patients for treatment their approach quickly becomes predictive of something unpleasant, increasing the likelihood the dog will show aggression to them. This can be avoided by incorporating interactions the dog enjoys into the treatment plan. The type of interaction needs to be tailored to the dog's condition, what they find pleasurable, and temperament. Examples include hand feeding part of the dog's ration or treats, grooming, fuss or massage. Even seemingly highly aggressive or fearful dogs can often be won over by tossing treats or kibble to the back of the kennel regularly throughout the day. Ideally, positive interactions will outweigh examinations and medical interventions by 3:1.

Environmental management

Effective air circulation will help remove stress pheromones that may affect other dogs. Ambient temperature should be maintained to prevent hyper- or hypothermia. Avoid bright artificial lighting when not immediately needed, to encourage dogs to rest.

Music

Research suggests classical music can reduce barking behaviour compared to talk radio, popular music or no additional sound. Heavy metal music is reported to increase barking.

9 Approach and Handling of the Patient

One of the greatest influences over the use of aggression in the practice is the approach and handling of the staff. Handling the dog in a way he will find uncomfortable is unavoidable at times for their welfare. However, there are a number of steps that can be taken to reduce any perceived threat in our handling and so reduce the likelihood he will react defensively (also see Chapter 10 for additional preventative handling of puppies and Appendix 2 for an information poster).

Know Your Patient

There are many potential influences over dog behaviour (see Chapter 2). The first step in preventing aggression is therefore to take a few minutes to get to know the temperament and usual behaviour of each individual dog before trying to interact with him. This is not as complex as it sounds.

Establish a routine of taking and recording a brief behavioural history of every dog attending the practice whether for a consultation or admission. An example patient behavioural assessment is given in Appendix 3. Assessment should involve both the owner's descriptions of behaviour and the observed behaviour during initial interactions. Methods for recording this information in the patient's record will vary according to computer system used. However, a simple code can usually be added to the patient's main clinical record so this is immediately highlighted, with more details of the assessment stored in sub-folders. An example scoring method for behaviour categories is given in Box 9.1.

Approach

Initial introduction

Avoid approaching, touching or staring at a dog when first meeting him. This applies to any first-time meeting, whether in the consulting room or the hospital. It is advisable to briefly explain to the client why you are doing this so they do not take offence. It is best to allow the dog to explore the new environment, whether having just entered a consulting room or been moved into a prep or other clinical area. If there are any concerns regarding the dog's safety he can be kept on lead and/or muzzled. However, there is a great deal to be gained by still allowing the dog a minute or two to explore the room and habituate to the new smells and objects before trying to handle or examine him.

Minor changes in current common practice can ensure this time is still productive. In the consultation room it can be used for taking the medical history and making the behavioural assessment. In the examination room it can be used to prepare equipment or read clinical notes. In both cases it can be used to assess the dog's current emotional state. This only takes a few seconds but can save a great deal of time and emotional distress for all concerned later. In particular, look for low-level signs of stress or threat, which, if recognized early, can enable steps to be taken before these escalate to more problematic behaviour (see Fig. 21).

Control emotional signals

Dogs are very intuitive to human emotions. Both owners and staff may be worried or fearful during an examination, or feeling the accumulated stress of a busy day. Whatever the reason for the human tension the dog will interpret this as a signal there is danger in the environment. It can therefore make a huge difference to the dog's behaviour if staff take a few seconds to calm themselves. Actively relaxing muscles and taking three or four slow deep breaths can release tension and clear the mind. Recognizing if a client is upset and taking steps to try and identify why and alleviating this can also be effective. In many cases simply giving them the opportunity to express their concern can dissipate it.

Let the dog set the pace

Allow the dog to approach and make contact with you in his own time rather than the other way around, where possible. Observe his body language as he does so. Most dogs will approach in a relaxed and confident way. However, even when they do so it is still important to avoid behaviour the dog may see as threatening. If the dog initiates contact pet him briefly under the chin or on the bib and then stop. Move your hand a few centimetres away and observe his response. If the dog is enjoying being petted he will try to re-initiate contact by moving forward, nuzzling your hand or showing social engagement behaviours.

If the dog seems relaxed, keen to interact and to be touched the examination can proceed following the principles in Table 37 and Figs 62–65. However, if the dog withdraws or shows signs of concern proceed as for nervous and reluctant dogs below.

It is good practice to get into the routine of handling all dogs in this way even if they are known to be friendly. This establishes doing so as your standard way of approaching and interacting with every dog. They will not eliminate a dog's fear completely. However, they will help reduce the factors pushing the dog closer to his bite threshold and also guard against those occasions when a normally friendly dog is worried or feeling defensive due to trigger stacking of unusual influences over his behaviour (see Part 2 and Fig. 60).

Ask any new people entering the room to also allow the dog to approach them in the same way and to adopt the same handling techniques. When rushed it is tempting for the new addition to simply get on with the job in hand. However, those few moments of introduction can save a great deal of time later trying to manage or placate an aggressive dog.

Nervous and reluctant dogs

If a dog seems worried the steps described in Table 37 can be expanded on with those in Table 38.

Box 9.1. Example method of scoring canine behaviour categories.

Situation code

A On arrival before making approach or contact
H When approached, examined or handled
I   During intervention

Behaviour code

1 Relaxed, friendly, no suggestion of concern
2 Low-level appeasing signals without withdrawal
3 Appeasing signals and withdrawal
4 Low-level threat: tension and posture only
5 Higher threat: growl, snarl, snap
6 Intense threat: lunging, snapping, bite history

Each dog is given a 6-digit code based on their behavioural response in each situation, e.g. A1 H3 I3

Table 37. Approach and handling of friendly dogs.

Principle	Description
Talk calmly	Talk quietly and calmly using the dog's name. This reduces the impression of threat.
Avoid leaning over	This mimics the 'standing over' threat posture dogs use at times of conflict. It can therefore be threatening and trigger a dog to react defensively. Be aware of the dog's personal space.
Approach at an angle	Dogs avoid walking directly towards each other when greeting as this is confrontational. Approaching from behind may take the dog by surprise. Approach from an angle but in clear line of sight.
Crouch down	Keep upright until you are close to the dog then turn so you are facing either at a 45° angle away from him or at his side facing the same direction as him, depending on what you need to do. Crouch down and look away as you do. Keep at least one foot flat on the ground so you can withdraw if needed.
Allow to greet	Allow him to explore the hand closest to him held loosely with fingers curled inwards about 10 cm away from your chest. Look to one side of the dog as you do so.
Touch under the chin or on the bib	Touching the back of a dog's neck can mimic the canine threat behaviour of one dog covering the other dog's neck with the head. Contact is therefore better under the chin or on the bib, once the dog is comfortable with you by his side.

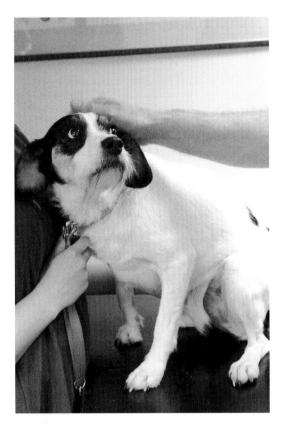

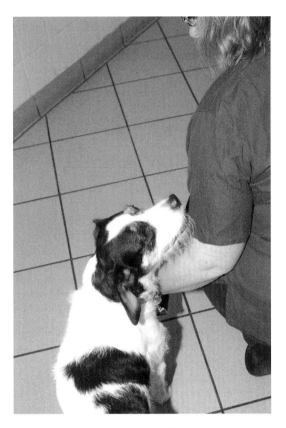

Fig. 62. A fearful dog in the vets. This dog is showing signs of significant fear at being on the table, the direct head-on approach and contact to the back of her head. This is seen in the crescent moon eye, clenched feet, ears pulled back and body weight cowering away. In some dogs this could escalate to aggression if the vet persists (see Fig. 35).

Fig. 63. Approach from the side. The change in approach here shows a completely different response. By allowing her to stay on the floor, approaching from the side and crouching down to her level she no longer feels threatened or afraid.

Removing a dog from a hospital cage

When handling a hospitalized dog the first point of contact is the approach to the cage. Following the principles summarized in Tables 37 and 38 will avoid causing the dog to feel concerned.

Where possible open the cage door and step to one side to allow the dog to step out voluntarily rather than reaching for, picking up or pulling the dog out. Staff can then approach from the side either standing up straight or crouching down to attach the lead as necessary. If the dog is nervous or allowing him outside of the cage off lead would be unsafe, a lead can be left on the dog whilst in the kennel. This must always be attached to a flat collar or harness (never a slip lead or check chain) and should not be tied to the cage door or any other

fixture to avoid the dog causing injury to himself, or becoming distressed or frustrated. If necessary link two or more leads together so they are long enough to be grasped from outside of the kennel using a traditional cat grabber. Once the lead is grasped step to one side and allow the dog to step out as above (see Fig. 66).

If a dog has had his lead removed and subsequently seems threatening or fearful in the kennel, make a large noose with a slip lead and slide it into the cage through a door held open a few inches. The dog will usually slide his head in as he tries to step out (see Fig. 67). The lead can then be tightened sufficiently to prevent removal but not tight enough to cause pain or make the dog fearful. If you cannot approach the dog to adjust the slip lead then a dog catcher/snare pole will need to be used (see below).

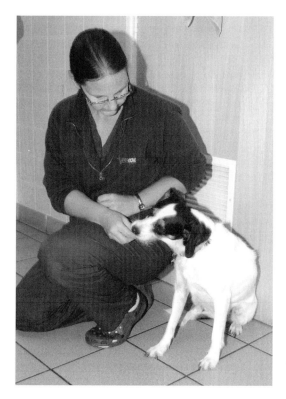

Fig. 64. Use of treats in handling. The side approach again helps her feel more comfortable. The addition of treats helps classically condition being in the practice to positive emotions, and rewards the decision to approach. However, care should be taken not to lure the dog closer than she is ready for with them.

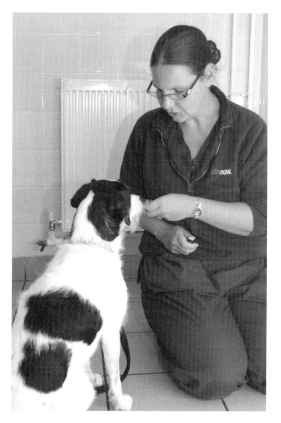

Fig. 65. Using training in handling can help. Some dogs relax when they are asked to perform and are rewarded for obeying commands as it offers them a clear way to behave they know leads to good outcomes.

Table 38. Additional considerations for handling a nervous or worried dog.

Positioning the dog	Ask the owner to move the dog to the centre of the room before approaching so you are not cornering him. Avoid standing between the dog and the door so you do not block his escape.
Avoid direct eye contact	Prolonged eye contact is threatening to a dog. It is therefore important to make a conscious effort to avoid doing so. Train yourself to look at the dog's ear or collar. Brief eye contact to read the dog's signals is acceptable but do not maintain this for more than a second.
Use dog calming signals	Try turning your head slightly, squinting or slow blinking, relaxing your mouth and moving your body weight away from the dog.
Avoid sudden movements	Dogs that are worried may react to any sudden movement. This will elevate the dog's stress levels and so potential for defensive behaviour.

Physical Manipulation

Physically manipulating a dog can cause distress in even the best natured and most confident dog. Pulling a dog towards you will force him into closer proximity than he may be comfortable with, without the option to withdraw. This can be sufficient to trigger higher level aggression. Many dogs are also fearful of being pulled by their collar, due to having been excessively manipulated by the collar or the collar being used to grab the dog for punishment in the

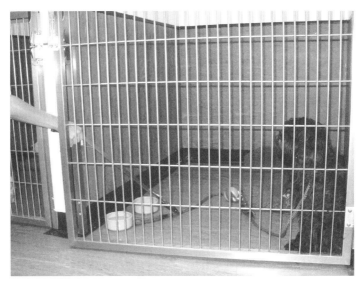

Fig. 66. Using a cat grabber to grasp a long lead in the kennel of an aggressive dog.

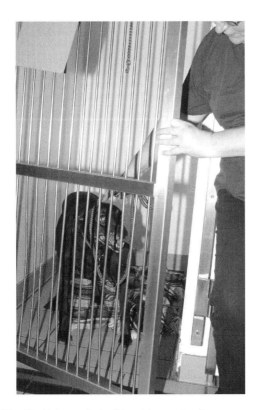

Fig. 67. Using a slip lead to retrieve a dog from a kennel. By standing to one side and positioning the noose of the slip lead by the exit the dog's head can be manipulated into it as he tries to leave.

past. As such, although the instinctive tendency is to use more restraint in a worried or threatening dog, this is counterproductive in many cases. It is therefore best avoided where possible.

Floor or table?

The decision whether to examine the dog on the floor or on a table needs to reflect both the size and temperament of the dog. Many dogs find being placed on a table worrying, especially if they are not familiar with it or have learnt to associate it with unpleasant procedures. Others may be completely comfortable with it. It is also hard not to loom over very small dogs on the floor and so putting them on a table will avoid this.

Check with the owner how familiar and comfortable the dog is with being on a table as part of the initial behavioural history taking. Test the dog's response wherever possible by lowering a hydraulic table and inviting the dog to get on. Lures can be used where appropriate, but if he seems distressed or chooses to get off as soon as he has eaten them it suggests he does not feel comfortable with it. In this case it is better to examine the dog on the floor. If small dogs seem worried by high tables they may feel more comfortable on a low sturdy box or square cat basket, enabling staff to handle them on the floor without looming over them.

Avoiding manipulation

Manipulation can be avoided by using commands or lures wherever possible to place the dog in the position needed. Treats or food stuffs can also be used to both engage and counter-condition dogs to certain treatments. However, it is critical that treats are not used to distract the dog and that he is fully aware of what is happening or he may suddenly become fearful when he notices. The aim is that he knows what you are doing but is more interested in the food. Examples of ways food can be used to engage the dog are given in Table 39.

Where a dog does not know a command and a lure is contraindicated or impractical, manipulation for the current examination may be unavoidable. This is generally best performed by the client, whom the dog is likely to be less worried by. If the client is unable or not present then aim to use manipulation techniques that minimize threat, support the body at all times and follow the dog's natural reflexes and postures. The safer and more natural the manipulation feels to the dog the less likely he is to resist it (see Figs 72–76). Continue to monitor body language and modify handling if the dog starts to show signs of concern. In most cases this will involve withdrawing and reassessing the approach. If the dog is nervous or seems mildly unsettled by the handling it may be better to apply a muzzle than to use greater restraint.

Clients can be encouraged to teach their dog to accept various forms of handling to prevent the need for manipulation on subsequent visits (see Chapter 10). Clients should be discouraged from using coercive training (see Chapter 7).

Safety first

It must be noted that these methods may not work for already highly aroused or aggressive dogs. They also don't eliminate all of a dog's concern at being in the practice. The aim is to be aware of ways in which changes in handling can avoid triggering higher levels of aggression or learn fear of visiting the practice. Where safety dictates short-term stronger restraint may still be unavoidable.

Equipment

Using muzzles

Muzzling is less stressful and less likely to provoke defensive behaviour than forced restraint. Therefore, when there is a choice between the two, muzzling is the preferred option.

Cage muzzles are preferable to cloth muzzles as they are generally better tolerated and allow the dog to pant for thermoregulation and to relieve stress. They also allow the dog to show normal appeasing behaviour such as licking his lips, yawning etc., which both provides the staff with ongoing information and prevents anxiety caused by inability to do so.

Short-term acceptance can be facilitated by smearing peanut butter or cream cheese inside the muzzle. The dog should be encouraged to voluntarily put his nose in to the muzzle rather than having it pushed on (see Fig. 77). Clients should be encouraged to familiarize the dog to wearing a muzzle at home for future visits. How to do so is outlined in Appendix 4.

Restraint equipment

Where circumstances dictate use of restraint equipment it is important that it is used correctly for safety, welfare and to prevent a traumatic experience that will make the dog more likely to behave defensively on subsequent occasions.

Table 39. Ways to use food to engage a dog.

Method	Description
Intra-nasal	Smear sticky foods such as cream cheese or peanut butter on the syringe for the dog to lick off or use a food lure to elevate the head (see Fig. 68).
Non IV injections	Place a number of small treats or smear a sticky food on to the table or floor in front of the dog for him to lick off as he is injected (see Fig. 69).
Foot examination	Hold a spoon with sticky food stuff to one side so the dog needs to turn his head away from the foot being treated (see Fig. 70).
Manners Minder	This is a remote delivery reward system that can be used to engage a dog during a prolonged treatment (see Fig. 71).
Toys or chews	Depending on the procedure and the dog's condition, chews or chew toys may be used to engage a dog during long procedures. This is not suited to possessive aggressive dogs.

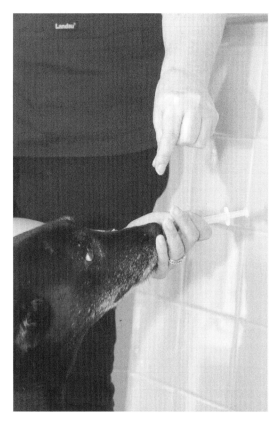

Fig. 68. Use of a food lure to entice a dog to raise his head for an intra-nasal vaccination.

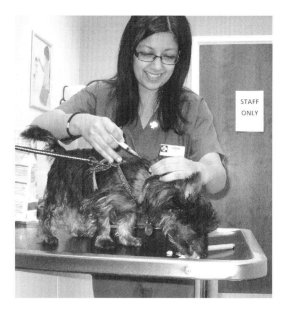

Fig. 69. Treats placed on the table can engage a dog for an injection into the scruff.

Clients should be asked to ensure their dog is wearing a properly fitted flat collar prior to admission and handling. The fitting and condition of the collar and lead can be visually assessed by asking the client to place two fingers under the collar, to try pulling the collar over the dog's head and to rotate the collar and hold out the lead so any damage or areas of weakness can be spotted. This minimizes the need for staff to have to fit collars or to use practice equipment for moving the dog around.

In some circumstances it will still be necessary to use practice equipment. The factors that should be taken into consideration when choosing suitable equipment are summarized in Table 40.

Dog catchers/snare poles must be properly functioning, incorporate a locking mechanism to prevent over (or under) tightening and a quick release mechanism. When adjusting the noose to fit, it should be no tighter than a standard collar. This will ensure the dog cannot escape without triggering

fear due to pain or a sensation of being asphyxiated. There is nothing to be gained by making the noose tighter than this. It must be kept in mind if a dog is restrained on a dog catcher his 'flight' option has been removed, increasing the possibility of 'fight'.

Responding to Aggression

If a dog shows threat signals these should be interpreted as a sign that the dog is fearful and wants to be left alone. It is therefore best for all concerned to do so initially and evaluate the options rather than press ahead with forced restraint that may be avoidable.

Allow the dog to calm

Once a dog has become highly stressed or defensive he is very likely to persist with trying to repel the perceived threat until it has gone or he reaches exhaustion. The effects of the acute 'fight or flight' response are relatively short lived, so taking the dog out of the stressful environment for a period of 15 min may enable him to calm so the examination can then be attempted again using a different approach. However, chronic stress lasts much longer and so if that has been triggered by a prolonged or intense struggle, or the dog was already stressed before the

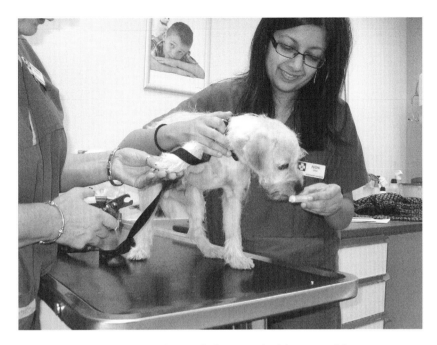

Fig. 70. Using sticky food to engage a dog during a nail clip can make it less stressful.

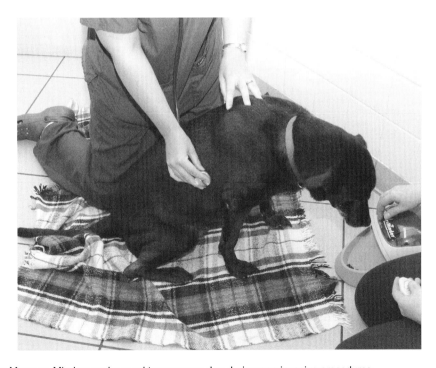

Fig. 71. The Manners Minder can be used to engage a dog during non-invasive procedures.

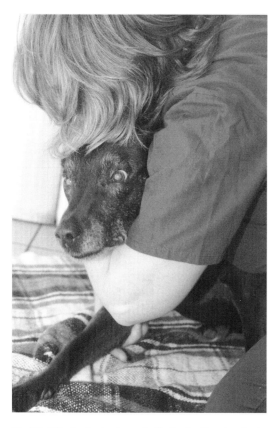

Fig. 72. This dog is clearly worried by the traditional methods of restraining, seen in his furrowed brow and staring eyes.

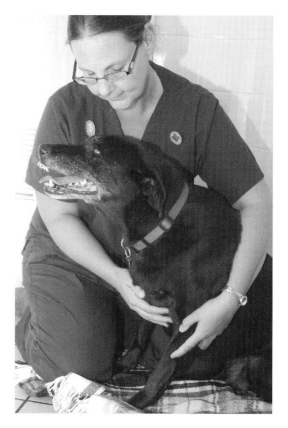

Fig. 73. An alternative approach for raising a vein. Here a gentler approach is adopted using light restraint on the front of the chest and the arm across the back to raise the vein instead of over the neck. The right hand is still in position to take a firmer grasp if needed. Where it is felt the dog's behaviour is unpredictable a cage muzzle can be applied for safety.

examination started, he may not calm in this time frame. He may also have learnt to expect conflict in this situation and so become defensive much more quickly. If this occurs the approach needs to be re-evaluated further (see below).

Postponing the consultation

Depending on the purpose of the visit it may be possible to postpone the consultation. This may allow time for the dog to calm sufficiently for re-examination. It may also provide an opportunity for the client to perform muzzle or handling training or for the dog to be counter-conditioned to visiting the practice or some procedures (see Table 42, Chapters 12 and 14, and Appendix 4).

In some cases re-arranging the consultation as a house visit may help by removing those triggers linked to the practice. Booking with a staff member of a different gender or appearance may also help if this is adding to the dog's triggers.

Depending on the problem, the veterinary surgeon may choose to forgo the examination by using trial therapies based on reported history, or may provide pain relief to remove the aggravatory trigger of pain. He or she may also decide to perform the examination under sedation or a general anaesthetic.

Medication

Short-acting anxiolytic medication may help reduce the likelihood of aggression in some cases. The effects of medication are discussed in Chapter 7. However, it must be borne in mind that when medication removes fear the resulting increase in confidence may occasionally increase the risk of aggression in some cases. This is not common but must be kept in mind.

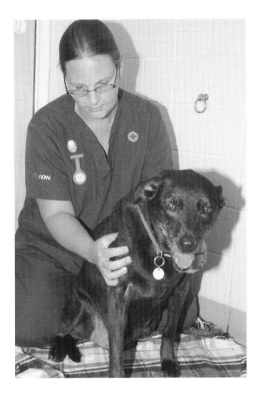

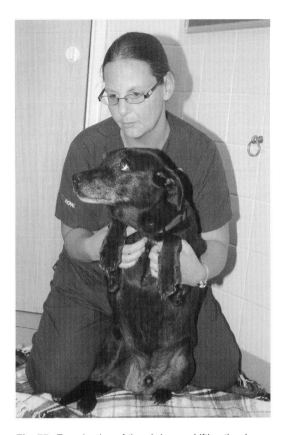

Fig. 74. An alternative approach for keeping still. If a dog needs to prevented from moving forwards or backwards he may feel more comfortable sitting between the nurse's or technician's legs with hands resting on the front of the chest. This handling does add to the dog's stress but allows for a firmer grip to be taken if needed. Again, use of a muzzle is advisable if the dog's behaviour is potentially unpredictable.

Fig. 75. Examination of the abdomen. Lifting the dog from the above seated position can enable examination of the ventral abdomen without needing to force the dog on to his side.

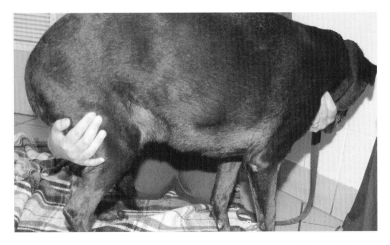

Fig. 76. Lowering into a sit. Dogs that do not know a sit command can be lowered into a sit by gently scooping under the hind limbs. This tends to meet with less resistance than attempting to push down on the back.

Approach and Handling of the Patient

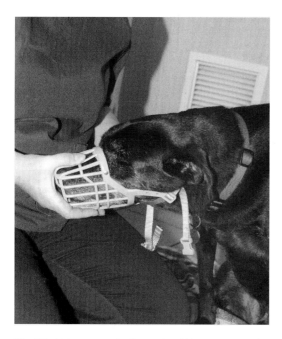

Fig. 77. Using a muzzle. Dogs should be encouraged to voluntarily put their nose into the muzzle rather than having it pushed on to their nose.

Table 40. Factors to consider when choosing practice restraint equipment.

Factor	Discussion
Ease of fitting	Equipment needs to be easy to put on, take off and adjust. Collars with plastic snap buckles are suitable.
Mode of action	Slip leads are convenient in practice but standard slip leads are aversive and potentially harmful. This effect can be prevented by moving the stopper to sit on the side of the slip ring closer to the neck (see Fig. 48) or by using slip leads with patented metal buckle sliders designed to prevent over tightening.
Hygiene	Unless collars and leads are disposable they must be easily disinfected.
Physiology and injury	Choice of equipment will vary according to the dog's shape. For example, standard flat neck collars can be easily slipped off by some dolichocephalic breeds. It may be hard to find a harness that will fit some shapes of dog. Consideration also needs to be given to any injuries, surgical wounds or disease such as to the neck or spine.

PART 3
Behavioural Prophylaxis

Veterinary nurses and technicians play many key roles in preserving life and ensuring animal welfare. One such area is ensuring owners receive prompt and accurate advice to enable them to prevent problem behaviour developing.

Primarily this will be when advising on how to raise puppies. Practice staff are there at the very start of the relationship between the responsible dog owner and their new puppy and so have a valuable role to play in ensuring clients have good quality advice and guidance from the outset. This applies equally to the first time puppy owner and the more experienced owner who may not be aware of relatively recent changes in our understanding of canine behaviour, handling and training methods. Practices can provide advice through puppy consultations, puppy socialization classes, practice literature, website features and waiting room displays. This both informs the client and bonds them to the practice.

Preventive behaviour advice can also be given in circumstances that carry a risk of leading to problem behaviour. For example, advising clients on how to settle in a rescue dog or manage the addition of a new family member, human or otherwise, can minimize these changes causing long-term problems. The potential behavioural impact of illness, injury or surgery can also be minimized with effective advice.

Finally, good advice can slow the behaviour effects of cognitive decline, support both client and patient during palliative care and help a remaining dog come to terms with the deterioration or loss of a companion.

10 Guidance for Puppy Owners

One of the first things many new puppy owners do is take their new addition to the vets. This will primarily be for an initial health check, vaccination and worming treatment. However, this contact also offers the opportunity to advise owners on behavioural management and training of their puppy. Research has shown that puppies given behavioural guidance in the veterinary practice show fewer problem behaviours such as house soiling, inappropriate mounting, mouthing and aggression to unfamiliar dogs and people (Gazzano *et al.*, 2008). Time spent offering such advice is therefore a worthwhile investment.

Experiences in the Practice

Positive associations lessen the development of negative ones. Ensuring that early experiences at the practice are positive will therefore go a long way to reducing problem behaviour during future visits. Chapters 8 and 9 discuss how to manage initial approaches and handling during veterinary visits. Box 10.1 gives further suggestions to meet the specific needs of puppies.

Prior to Adoption

Puppies are typically adopted by their new owners between 7 and 9 weeks of age. As such they spend the majority of their sensitive period for socialization and habituation with the dam and siblings, and under the care of the breeder/dam's owner. The veterinary practice is in an excellent position to ensure that any of their clients that breed dogs are up to date with best practice for providing for their puppies' behavioural development.

Mating, pregnancy and parturition

Maternal stress can affect the ability of offspring to cope with stressors (see Chapter 2). Breeders can minimize the likelihood of this by ensuring the mating, pregnancy and parturition are as stress free as possible. Tips for doing so are summarized in Box 10.2.

If the dam needs to be induced this is best performed during a home visit to minimize stress around the time of parturition. If this is not possible she should be sent home again straight after the injection has been administered.

If a caesarean section is indicated the dam should be admitted to a quiet area of the practice for as short a period as possible prior to surgery. A collapsible covered crate in a non-clinical area can be utilized if there are no quiet kennels available. The behavioural effects of surgery can be minimized as outlined in Box 10.3.

If the dam does not survive, is incapable of caring for or rejects the puppies it will be important to provide for their behavioural as well as their physical needs. Ideally a surrogate dam will be found but this is not always possible. If the puppies have to be hand reared extra care will need to be given to ensure they receive adequate socialization to other dogs. How to do this is discussed below.

Socialization and habituation

The principles of the canine sensitive periods of socialization and habituation are discussed in Chapter 2. The effects of poor social and environmental experiences during this period must not be underestimated. Breeders therefore have a responsibility to ensure their puppies have appropriate experiences during this critical time.

Socialization to people

Gentle human handling from birth familiarizes the puppy to human scent and starts development of appropriate responses to mild stressors (see Box 10.4). Once the puppies can see and hear they should also

Box 10.1. Creating positive associations to the practice for puppies.

- Place a few treats on the table then ask the client to place the puppy on so he finds them waiting when he gets there.
- Provide washable toys to direct puppy attention and redirect mouthing.
- Use treats or food paste smeared on to scales to lure the puppy on to them.

- Drop a few treats on the table and allow the puppy to eat them as injections are given.
- Arrange for additional visits when there are no procedures planned.
- Arrange puppy socialization classes at the practice (see Chapter 11).

Box 10.2. Steps to reduce maternal stress.

- Allow the dam and sire to mate naturally. Avoid forced mating, muzzling or excessive interference.
- Allow the bitch to stay in her familiar environment. Moving house, rehoming or moving the bitch to a different location for her pregnancy are best avoided.

- Protect the bitch against stressful events. Provide refuge or support if these occur unavoidably, e.g. thunderstorms (see Chapter 14).
- Avoid stressing the bitch during parturition. Provide a quiet area and supervise unobtrusively.

Box 10.3. Minimizing the behaviour effects of caesarean section.

- Impregnate a clean cloth with the dam's scent by wiping it over the mammary area prior to preparation for surgery. Place in a sealed plastic bag to preserve the scent.
- Prepare a suitable quiet kennel or covered crate for after surgery. Line with clean blankets plus a single blanket from the bitch's own bed.
- The area surrounding the incision site should be routinely cleaned post-surgery then washed

with plain warm water to remove all residue of skin disinfectants. Allow to dry then use the cloth prepared above to re-establish the dam's normal scent by wiping it over the mammary area but avoid the wound itself.
- Place the puppies in a box near to the dam as she recovers from the anaesthetic. Supervise her around them until she is steady on her feet and actively caring for and nursing them.

Box 10.4. Gentle handling of newborn puppies for socialization and development of stress responses.

- Start at 3 days of age.
- Each puppy should be handled daily for about 2 min. This is best performed at times when they are calm and not hungry.
- The puppy should be gently supported throughout handling.

- The tummy and feet should be gently stroked and ears gently rubbed.
- All handling must be slow, gentle and calm.
- If the puppy seems distressed the client should stop and try again later. The aim is to gently familiarize the puppy to human handling, not to trigger higher levels of stress.

---

have the opportunity to meet and be handled by a variety of people so they become socialized to people of different genders, skin colours, appearance and ages. People visiting the house to help socialize the puppies should be asked to remove outdoor footwear and coats and to wash their hands before entering the puppies' pen. They should get down to the puppies' level and allow the dam and puppies to approach and initiate interactions. They can then fuss the puppies as they normally would or allow them to climb on their lap. All contact should be calm and gentle but the way in which the puppies are fussed or greeted should only be limited by the puppies' responses. Some forms of human handling may be contrary to how dogs normally interact. Touching on the back of the head or neck can be a threat if performed by one dog to another. However, this is a very common way for people to greet or fuss a dog. As such, familiarizing the puppy to this during their sensitive period can guard against them seeing this as worrying when it inevitably happens in later life. Children allowed to fuss the puppies must be well behaved and old enough to follow direction from supervising adults. Younger children can be allowed to watch the puppies from outside the pen or play alongside them on the other side of a barrier.

Socialization to other dogs

Puppies ordinarily develop olfactory recognition of other dogs via their dam and/or siblings. If a puppy is orphaned it is important to compensate for this by exposing him to dog odours, either by being in the same room as other vaccinated dogs or by using scented cloths.

The puppies will develop social skills during play with their siblings and interactions with the dam. Play should be monitored and bullying or excessive control of one puppy over another interrupted (see Chapter 5). Excessive corrections by the dam should also be prevented.

Puppies should be given multiple feeding bowls when weaning to prevent excessive competition, which may encourage possessive behaviour later

in life. The puppies should also have access to multiple toys and chews for the same reason.

Household sounds

Puppies should be exposed to a range of household sounds from around 2–3 weeks of age. These should include those that may trigger a stress response in later life, e.g. the washing machine, vacuum cleaner, lawn mower or hair dryer. Puppies bred outdoors or in isolated rooms in the house, such as a breeding room, utility or conservatory, are at particular risk of not habituating to these sounds and so need to be actively exposed to them on a daily basis.

Naturally occurring stimuli are the most effective. However, these are not always practical. Where natural stimuli are not available the use of artificial stimuli such as sound and video recordings have been shown to be at least partially effective. This method is particularly useful for exposure to sounds that are out of the breeder's control such as thunder, fireworks and gunshot.

Choosing a Puppy

Most clients acquire their puppy without making any prior contact with the surgery. However, some may approach the practice for advice on what type of puppy to get or where to get the puppy from.

Choosing the right type of dog

Table 41 summarizes the behavioural considerations to be taken into account when choosing the right type of puppy for them.

Table 41. Behavioural factors to consider when choosing what type of puppy to adopt.

Factor	Discussion
Breed	Clients need to research which breed best matches the amount of exercise, mental stimulation, training and companionship they are able to provide. A mismatch is one of the key reasons for problem behaviour. They should never choose a breed on looks alone (see Chapter 3).
Space	Larger dogs physically need more space. Less sociable dogs also need space to retreat to and thought must be given to space when introducing new dogs into a multi-dog household. The proximity of neighbours needs to be considered when acquiring commonly vocal or territorial breeds.
Toilet training	Effective toilet training requires access to an enclosed outside space that will not be frequented by unvaccinated dogs. If the client only has access to a communal garden it may be possible to arrange for a section to be temporarily partitioned off and covered with a new substrate until vaccinations are complete.

Evaluating the source of the puppy

It is important the clients acquire their puppy from a reliable source. Many dogs with behavioural problems originated from irresponsible breeders and puppy farms. Deprived and isolated environments can be highly detrimental to a puppy's development by interfering with normal socialization, habituation and development of the ability to cope with stress. Impoverished conditions also often lead to illness, which can further negatively impact on development as the puppy has to be nursed back to health.

Accredited breeder schemes help identify those breeders that have taken the care to register with them. Puppy contracts can also provide valuable information when assessing the care the breeder takes. Although these are useful clients should be advised to also perform their own checks to ensure the chosen scheme is robust and the breeder is actually adhering to its requirements. Box 10.5 summarizes the key things to look for when evaluating a puppy source.

Clients also need to be aware that many unscrupulous puppy 'traders' can be quite elaborate in their methods of hiding their true breeding and rearing practices. Excuses for not allowing prospective owners to view the puppies at home with the dam need to be explored and verified. Clients should be warned against ploys such as delivering the puppy direct to the client's home to be helpful or being promised a chance to meet the dam, which then evaporates when they arrive due to an 'emergency'. Clients should be actively encouraged to report any suspicious breeders to the relevant authorities.

If suspicion is not triggered until the puppy is in their arms many clients will find it hard to then reject it. Such clients often need to visit the practice early due to generally poor condition. This provides the practice with an opportunity to direct the client to an accredited behaviourist early so steps can be taken to minimize the effects of these early experiences. Ensure clients realize time is of the essence when doing so.

Post-adoption

The transition

Adoption day will be exciting for the new owners but is a traumatic experience for the puppy. Every step must therefore be taken to minimize the negative impact of this and help the puppy settle in quickly and easily. Key points to consider are summarized in Box 10.6.

Introductions

In most cases the puppy will already have been introduced to other animal members of the household by the time he reaches the practice. However, some clients may seek advice prior to doing so. The advice in Boxes 10.7, 10.8 and 10.9 is intended for introducing the puppy to existing dogs, cats and other small animals that show no concern around dogs. However, this may not always be the case. Owners need to understand that existing pets may not automatically share their enthusiasm for the new puppy. If there is any doubt or an existing dog already has problems the client should be referred to an accredited behaviourist so the prognosis for the puppy being accepted can be discussed and any existing problems resolved before trying to do so.

Box 10.5. Things to look for when evaluating a puppy source.

- Check the breeder considers the behaviour and temperament of the dam and the sire when choosing from which individuals to breed.
- Ask what steps are taken to minimize stress during mating, pregnancy and parturition.
- Check the puppies are kept with the dam and allowed to suckle unimpeded.
- Check the puppies are handled regularly in a calm, structured way.

- Check the puppies are reared in the communal part of the house or are brought into this area regularly for habituation if they are bred outdoors or in separate breeding rooms .
- Ask to meet the dam at the same time as the puppies. Check she is of a relaxed and friendly disposition both inside and outside of the house.
- Choose a puppy that approaches new people and welcomes their attention.

Box 10.6. Steps to ease a puppy's transition from breeder to new home.

- The breeder should be asked to provide cloths impregnated with the dam's scent that can be placed with the puppy during the journey and in his bed at the new home. If necessary the new owner can give these to the breeder to place in the nest a few days before collection.
- The puppy should be placed in a crate with lots of soft bedding for the journey home. The crate should be either secured by seatbelt or in the boot. The puppy should have access to water for all but the briefest of journeys.

- Use of Adaptil™ spray in the car and diffusers by the puppy's bed can help ease the initial transition.
- The client should be advised to avoid any new experiences other than meeting the immediate family and the change of home for the first few days so as not to overwhelm the puppy.
- How to introduce the puppy to existing animal residents is discussed below.
- Changes in diet should not be made for the first few weeks, unless the existing diet is deficient in some way. Changes should be made gradually.

Box 10.7. Steps for introducing a new puppy to an existing dog.

- Someone should take the existing dog for a walk before the new puppy arrives.
- The puppy should be taken into the garden to eliminate on arrival.
- The puppy should be allowed to explore the house under supervision.
- The puppy should be shown his crate and fed something interesting in it.
- Once he has finished, the crate door can be closed but the client should stay with him. The existing dog can then be brought into the room and the dogs allowed to greet through the bars.
- If they are relaxed with each other the puppy can then be allowed out of the crate. A trailing line is best left on the existing dog initially so he can be calmly led away if needed.
- The older dog should be provided with a bed or refuge the puppy cannot reach so he can withdraw if he wants to.

- The client should spend quality time alone with each dog. This prevents the existing dog being pushed out and ensures the puppy bonds with the owner as well as the other dog.
- Play should be supervised to ensure the existing dog is neither too rough or too tolerant. The new puppy needs to learn acceptable social and play behaviour towards other dogs, so the owner will need to intervene if the adult dog allows the puppy to interact rudely or bully.
- The puppy should be confined to a crate when leaving the dogs alone so he can rest and to prevent excessive play.
- The dogs should initially be fed either side of a baby gate. The adult dog's ration can be spread over the same number of meals as the puppy.
- The puppy must spend brief periods without the other dog so he gets used to this.

On-going socialization and habituation

Once the puppy is in his new home the breeder's socialization and habituation programme should be continued and expanded.

Other dogs

Continued social interaction with other dogs is absolutely essential but sadly often neglected. Puppies continue learning social skills such as greeting and play until maturity. Therefore they need to be given the opportunity to do so on a regular basis throughout their development. They also need to meet dogs that are markedly different to themselves, which they may not have had the opportunity to do at the breeders. This helps them feel comfortable with dogs that vary in size, colour, temperament and play behaviour.

The client should be encouraged to attend puppy socialization classes at the practice, puppy training classes run by accredited trainers and to arrange play dates. Social interactions should include dogs at different life stages. Puppies learn through play with other puppies, and learn rules and boundaries

Box 10.8. Steps for introducing a new puppy to an existing cat.

- The puppy and cat should be kept separate for the first few days.
- Place cloths in both the cat's and puppy's beds and swap them daily so they can get used to each other's scents.
- The puppy and cat should initially be allowed to meet whilst the puppy is quietly eating a stuffed Kong or similar in his crate.
- The cat should not be forced into the same room but the client can try enticing with some especially smelly and desirable food such as warm pilchards.
- These introductions should be repeated twice a day for 3 days.
- If the cat seems comfortable in the puppy's presence the client can start to let the puppy out of the crate for brief periods whilst the cat is there. The puppy should be on a trailing house lead so he can be calmly led away if needed. The cat must have an escape via a cat flap the puppy will not fit through, on to a high surface or behind a baby gate.
- The puppy should be distracted from any signs of chase behaviour.
- Never punish either the puppy or the cat for chase or defensive behaviour.
- As they relax, periods spent together can be gradually increased until they no longer need to be specifically supervised. However, it is important to maintain the above safe escapes for the cat lifelong and to ensure the cat always has access to a safe indoor place away from the puppy. Use of a Feliway in this space will help worried cats. It is also important to make sure the dog does not block the cat's access to these or to his/her food, water and litter trays.

Box 10.9. Steps for introducing a new puppy to existing small furries.

- Where the small furry is kept caged all the time or exercised away from the puppy, he can be taken to the small furry's cage and played with alongside it.
- If the small furry is allowed to roam free in the house or garden introductions can be made as for cats above.

---

from well-behaved older dogs. They therefore need supervised exposure to both. The puppy should only be exposed to fully vaccinated dogs until his own vaccinations are complete. How to manage interactions between two puppies is discussed in Chapter 11. When introducing a puppy to an adult dog, start with both on lead. If greeting is positive and relaxed they can then be let off lead (if in an enclosed area), but ensure both have the opportunity to withdraw if they want to and supervise play to ensure neither becomes pushy, over-excited or defensive.

As the puppy grows up and starts to have off-lead exercise he can also be encouraged to play with other good-tempered dogs met on walks. However, it is good practice for the client to initially recall the puppy and ask the other dog's owner if their dog is friendly towards other dogs or puppies before allowing free interaction. This reduces the chance he will try and greet an unsociable dog and also gets him into the habit of coming back to the owner before doing so. How to supervise play behaviour is discussed in Chapters 5 and 11.

Other species

It is important to expose the puppy to any other species he may need to behave acceptably with in the future. This may include species the client anticipates keeping as pets such as cats, rabbits, birds and small pet rodents. It also includes species he may encounter on walks, such as livestock, horses and wildlife.

Modes of transport

The puppy needs to learn not to be concerned in all forms of motorized transport. He should therefore be taken on car rides, even if the client does not drive, and on public transport such as buses and trains. The puppy can be made to feel more comfortable by being placed in a cat carrier with one of his own blankets and a toy, or by being carried. Adaptil™ spray can also be used (see Chapter 7).

Different environments

Puppies need to be exposed to different environments, especially those that differ from where he normally lives. This could include taking country dogs to the city and vice versa to prevent fear of busy places or open spaces.

Managing exposure

All socialization and habituation needs to be managed to ensure that the puppy's experiences are positive so they build rather than undermine confidence.

New stimuli should be introduced gradually. Only introduce one new stimulus at a time and start with each in a 'diluted' form, e.g. at a distance or from behind a screen.

It is important that the client observes and responds to the puppy's reactions to triggers. If he seems comfortable he should be allowed to explore in his own time. If he seems unsure the owner or a helper can show him that the stimulus is safe and fun by exploring it themselves. They should not try to lure him to go towards the stimulus as this may push him to go closer than he feels comfortable and then cause him to suddenly spook strongly and so become more fearful of the trigger. However, if he chooses to go closer and is relaxed around the stimulus he can be rewarded with treats or play.

The puppy should be given the chance to withdraw if he seems worried. This is how confidence is built. If he experiences something worrying but feels he can cope with it by retreating to somewhere safe he will start to learn not be afraid of it. If he meets something new and is unable to escape this will intensify his fear and make him more reluctant to approach again in the future. If he does withdraw he should be given time to decide for himself to try again. If he chooses to try again but still seems wary the client can then call him back for a treat, then allow him to explore once more.

The client should avoid making extra fuss of him when he is worried, to avoid any suggestion there is a reason to be. They should also avoid ignoring him as withdrawal of attention is a form of punishment and so could aggravate his anxiety around the stimulus. They should simply relax and act as if there is nothing odd going on. If the puppy does not want to approach or is strongly fearful they should withdraw and try again another day.

The chart in Appendix 5 provides a quick reference planner that will enable clients to ensure their puppy is given adequate exposure to a wide variety of stimuli over the remainder of the socialization and habituation period. Clients should also be made aware that whilst this period is the most sensitive for habituation, this needs to be continued throughout the puppy's development to ensure it does not regress and to allow continued development and confidence building.

Compensating for negative experiences

The older the puppy is the greater the frequency and duration of exposure needed for habituation to take place. Therefore whilst triggers that the puppy is already familiar with just need to be continued, new triggers, especially where the puppy had a deprived early start, need to be more frequent and longer to compensate for this.

If a puppy has a bad experience the first or first few times he experiences a trigger the owner must be prepared to actively compensate for it. They should follow the principles above but ensure that the trigger is sufficiently diluted for the puppy to show no concern at all towards it. They should repeat this exposure a few times, linked to something positive such as food or a game, before increasing the concentration of the trigger. If the worry persists the client should be advised to seek help from an accredited behaviourist.

Toilet Training

Effective toilet training is achieved through early classically conditioned associations between the sensations of being outdoors and elimination. The puppy is at his most sensitive for making this association between 7 and 9 weeks, as he will naturally start to seek elimination away from the nest at this time. To achieve classical conditioning of elimination outside, the puppy needs to be taken outside whenever he is likely to want to do so. The principal steps for toilet training a puppy are summarized in Box 10.10.

Ideally the puppy should not be left alone for longer than he can manage without needing to eliminate, other than overnight. This can be built up as his ability to hold urine grows. Clients should be advised to ignore elimination that occurs indoors. They must not punish him for earlier accidents as this may cause anxiety or confusion, or teach the puppy to hide the next time he needs to go, making toilet training harder. The mess can be cleaned up once the puppy has moved away and is distracted. The area should be thoroughly cleaned with a biological detergent. Advise the client to avoid ammonia-based cleaners as these smell very similar to urine and so can mark the area as a latrine to the puppy. If the puppy repeatedly urinates in one place advise the client to try moving his food or water bowls to the spot or, if necessary, block the puppy's access to that spot until he is fully toilet trained. Advise clients to avoid using newspaper or puppy pads as these encourage indoor elimination.

Teaching puppy to ask to go outside

Toilet training can sometimes be slowed because the puppy is asking to go into the garden but no-one notices. It can therefore be useful to teach a puppy to ask the client to open the door in a way that can be heard from anywhere in the house. This can be achieved by teaching the puppy to bark or to ring a bell (see Boxes 10.11 and 10.12).

Being Alone

Problem behaviour when a dog is left alone is common. There can be many causes for the behaviour, including that the dog has never learnt to feel

---

Box 10.10. Toilet training a puppy.

- The puppy should be taken out whenever it is likely he will want to eliminate, e.g. on waking, after eating or a period of play, before being left or when he starts to sniff and circle. Initially leave a gap of no more than 2 h between visits outside. It can help to keep a diary of the puppy's elimination behaviour in the first week or so to help identify patterns.
- Owners should avoid talking to or interacting with their puppy until he has eliminated as this will distract him.
- As he eliminates they should say a command word, e.g. 'do business'. This will teach him to associate the word with the action.
- An operant aspect to housetraining can be added by rewarding the puppy immediately after he has finished.

- If the puppy has not eliminated within 5 min they should bring him back in and try again later based on the guidelines above.
- If the puppy will be left alone for more than 15 min he should be restricted to an area he will not want to foul, e.g. his crate or feeding area.
- If the puppy is sleeping upstairs at night, toilet training will be speeded up if the owner also takes him out when he stirs in the night.
- As the puppy learns the command word this can be used to ask him to eliminate before being left.
- As accidents become fewer or stop, the length of time between each outside visit can be gradually increased.

Box 10.11. Teaching a puppy to bark to ask to go outside.

- The puppy should be shown a treat or favourite toy. This is then placed on the other side of the door, and the door is closed.
- The client should wait whilst the puppy tries different tactics to get them to open the door.
- As soon as the puppy barks the client should open the door to let the puppy have the treat or toy.
- If the puppy does not do so within about a minute he should be distracted away from the door with a different treat without opening the door. This step is most effective if it is performed by someone else.

- This should be repeated three or four times a day until the puppy consistently gives the right signal first time.
- Once the puppy has learned that barking will get his owner to open a door he may also try barking for other things too. As long as the owner does not give them to him this will quickly pass.
- If the puppy seems to find it hard to work out what to do even after a number of sessions or is not very vocal, teaching him to ring a bell may be more effective (see Box 10.12).

---

comfortable on his own. This can be prevented by teaching the puppy to gradually accept being left on his own from a young age.

Very young puppies naturally want to stay close to a care giver for protection. As they start to grow up they become more willing to wander further and to spend time alone, as long as it is in a 'safe' place. The age at which the puppy starts to feel comfortable doing so is still being researched. Elliot and Scott (1961) showed that distress vocalizations in a strange place were greatest at about 7 weeks of age. They also found that puppies left alone for the first time at 12 weeks showed strong distress. Another study suggested that puppies show less stress when left once they are over 90 days of age or have been in the new owner's possession for more than 6 days (Frank *et al.*, 2007). Both studies suggest heightened distress at being left alone is due to a combination of age and the familiarity of the surroundings. It is therefore suggested puppies are allowed to get used to the place in which they will be left for at least a week before being gradually taught to accept being alone (by day or night) as outlined in Box 10.13.

Crate training

Using crates to manage puppy behaviour has become very common over the last 20 years. Teaching a puppy to accept being confined to a crate reduces the likelihood of elimination in the house, the risk of injury and of damage to valuable household items. Research shows that puppies left alone in a crate are no more distressed than puppies left alone outside of it (Frank *et al.*, 2007). However, whilst they can have their uses, excessive use or use for owner convenience rather than for safety or

---

Box 10.12. Teaching a puppy to ring a bell to ask to go outside.

- The client should install a bell by the door at a height the puppy can reach, e.g. a parrot bell, Christmas bell or traditional coiled doorbell.
- A little peanut butter, cream cheese or other food paste should be smeared on the bell.
- As the puppy licks it off the owner should say 'bell'.
- This should be repeated 4/5 times 3 times a day for 2–3 days.
- The client should then take the puppy to the bell and show him a treat and say 'bell'. When he touches the bell the client should give him the treat. Advise the client to be patient if he does

- not do so straight away. However, if he does not do so after a few minutes they should go back a step.
- This should be repeated 4/5 times 3 times a day for 2–3 days.
- Once he can obey this command reliably it can be used to ask him to ring the bell before being let into the garden. He will then choose to ring the bell to ask to go out.
- Once learnt, the puppy may use the bell to ask for other things too. As long as he isn't given them this will quickly pass.

Box 10.13. Teaching a puppy to accept being left alone.

- The client should start by leaving when the puppy is tired, well fed and has just been out into the garden.
- He should be placed in a safe place, such as his crate or a puppy-proofed area of the house.
- The puppy should be given something engaging such as a new toy or food item.
- The client should leave calmly but must not sneak away – it is important that the puppy knows he or she has gone.
- The puppy should be left for 5 min. The client should make sure he or she is somewhere the puppy cannot hear, see or smell them.
- The client should come back in regardless of what is happening, e.g. barking or whining.

- If the puppy is being quiet he can be greeted immediately.
- If he is making noise he should be asked to 'sit' then given attention. He should not be ignored for long periods as this is punishing.
- This should be repeated three to four times a day.
- The duration the puppy is left for should be increased by 5 min increments, up to 30 min, then 10 min increments up to an hour. Each increment should be repeated three or four times. As the duration he is left for goes up, the frequency can reduce.
- Even puppies that live with another dog must learn to be alone.

---

training can result in bored, frustrated and poorly behaved puppies. Guiding clients in correct use is therefore essential.

When the owner is at home crates should only be used for very short periods. They can be useful if the client needs to use the bathroom, is cooking or performing a task that means they cannot properly supervise the puppy for a few minutes, e.g. vacuum cleaning. However, placing the puppy in a crate for long periods whilst the owner is at home means the puppy is not being properly stimulated and misses opportunities to teach the puppy the right way to behave. Every opportunity missed to kindly teach him what to do is another step towards an unruly and unhappy adolescent or adult dog. Owners also need to recognize that each puppy has a given need for exercise or stimulation. The more time he spends in the crate the more he will need to pack into the brief periods he is out, intensifying the arousal level and impulsivity of his behaviour.

Periods spent in the crate whilst the owner is out should not exceed more than a few hours. Leaving a puppy in a crate for longer than he can manage without eliminating will cause him to soil the crate, which may lead to a breakdown in his natural desire not to soil his bed. This can make toilet training harder. See above regarding the age at which the puppy can start to be left alone at home.

Crates can offer a very good place of security, rest and escape for puppies that lack confidence by providing an 'escape to safety' (see Chapter 7).

Learning that the crate is a place of refuge keeps the nervous dog's 'flight' option open to him and so reduces the likelihood of threat or aggression. They also provide a clear place of refuge from children in the mind of both the puppy and the child from a very young age.

The puppy should stop being confined to the crate once he is toilet trained and has stopped behaviours that could cause him injury such as chewing. However, the crate can continue to be available with the door propped open if the puppy is settled sleeping in it or retiring to it when he wants to rest. Crates should never be used to isolate the puppy if he has done something the owner wants to deter repetition of.

Box 10.14 summarizes the key considerations for using a crate during puppy training.

Playpens

Playpens offer more room and space for play when not being supervised. If the puppy is to sleep downstairs his crate can also be placed inside a playpen with the door open at night, so he can leave the crate to eliminate if needed.

Managing Puppy Behaviour

Chewing and stealing

Chewing is part of the 'dissection' aspect of canine hunting behaviour. It is therefore normal. If a dog's

---

Box 10.14. The key considerations for using a crate for puppy training.

- The crate should be placed somewhere the puppy can get to at any time.
- The crate should be covered on all but one side. Advise the client to make sure the puppy will not overheat.
- A cloth from the dam's bed can be added initially. After a few days this can be swapped for a cloth the owner has worn or slept with.
- The puppy can be given two blankets that are washed in rotation, so he always has his own familiar smell while maintaining hygiene.
- The client should offer treats and special toys in the crate to make it a positive place to be.
- The puppy should be familiarized to the crate when someone is there before locking him in when he is alone.

- The puppy should never be punished in his crate or put there for 'time outs'.
- The puppy should not be locked in the crate for longer than he can manage without eliminating or for long periods.
- Children and visitors must be taught this is the puppy's place of refuge and so should not bother him if he goes in to rest or get away.
- The puppy should only be in the crate for very brief periods when the owner is there: this is time for learning about life.
- The puppy should stop being confined to his crate as soon as he is toilet trained and has stopped chewing. It can be kept as an open-door sleeping place as long as the puppy likes it.

---

normal daily ration does not require chewing the behaviour will be directed on to other things such as bones, toys, sticks or maybe the owner's personal possessions if there is nothing else. Although a certain amount of chewing is to be expected lifelong, there are usually periods of heightened chewing during puppy development. The first period occurs in very young puppies as they explore the world using their mouths. They tend to pick up and possibly chew on anything new they find to learn more about its texture, taste and edibility. Those that do not taste very nice or are boring will then be ignored in future, whereas things that are fun or satisfying to chew on will continue to be chewed. There are further periods of heightened chewing when the puppy is teething and as he reaches about a year of age.

Stealing food is also normal behaviour. Dogs are scavengers and so unattended food is a legitimate food source to them. Stealing non-edible items usually arises as an extension of chewing. The puppy starts by picking up an item to explore or play with. If he finds doing so is a very successful way to draw the owner's attention, he then starts picking up things as a way (in his mind) to incite the owner to play

'chase' games or to otherwise interact with him/her, perhaps at times when other play incitements are not successful.

Chewing can be managed by providing suitable things to chew to satisfy this drive and by ensuring the things the owner wants the puppy to chew on are the most fun and most satisfying. Stealing food is managed by keeping food not intended for the puppy or dog out of reach. Stealing other things can be prevented by ensuring the puppy does not see doing so as the best way to get the owner to interact with him.

Given that chewing and stealing are both normal behaviours they should never be punished. Inappropriate punishment for chewing and stealing, or forced removal of items is a common trigger for pre-emptive defensive aggression in later life.

How to prevent and manage chewing and stealing is summarized in Box 10.15.

Play

Play is an important part of puppy development. Puppies learn social skills, how to direct their hunting behaviour and how to control their impulses

---

Box 10.15. How to prevent and manage puppy stealing and chewing.

- The puppy should be provided with suitable toys for chewing. The nature of the toy will depend on breed and age but should include things that can be ripped up such as home-made treat toys.
- The puppy should be given access to two or three items at a time. These can be rotated or replaced daily to keep them interesting.
- Safe smells such as vanilla, aniseed and mint can be added to toys to keep them interesting.
- The client can carry or sleep with soft toys to impregnate them with human scent.
- The client should play interactive games with them to increase their interest compared to other things.
- Hard toys can be smeared with cream cheese, meat paste or other strong tasting/smelling food stuffs.
- The client should avoid letting a puppy chew things that can be confused with things he should not chew, e.g. old shoes.
- The client should put things it is important the puppy does not chew, whilst he is learning, out of reach. Supervise to ensure the puppy does not eat pieces he has chewed off.

- The puppy should be taught 'leave' and 'give' early on (see Appendix 6).
- If the puppy chews on or steals something he should not have a 'give' command can be used to retrieve it. He can then be given something else. This behaviour is a sign he is bored and so he must be given something to do.
- If he refuses to release the item the owner can try playing with another toy with someone else or on his or her own, or try scattering a few treats on the floor away from the puppy then covering the item with a cloth once he is distracted.
- The client should avoid chasing or tugging to remove the item. If the puppy will not relinquish easily it is best to walk away and ignore him for a few minutes. The item should only be forcibly removed if it is something he could seriously injure himself on.
- The puppy should never be punished for chewing.
- The client should be advised to see an accredited behaviourist as soon as possible if the puppy starts to become growly over possessions.

---

and their bite though play. Play also occupies a lot of a puppy's time and puppies that don't have enough opportunity to play are more likely to get into mischief.

Play should not be excessively regulated or controlled but should be monitored and directed if necessary. It can also be used as an opportunity for impulse control. Provide suitable toys for the puppy's age and breed and rotate these or change the smell of them to keep them interesting. If a puppy is behaving in an unwanted way, such as stealing, chewing things he should not have or trying to get attention through undesirable behaviour, it should be seen as a sign that the puppy is bored or his normal drives are not being fulfilled. The owner then needs to look at what exercise and stimulation the puppy is getting and modify them if needed.

Chase

Chase behaviour is a natural part of the canine hunting pattern. Many dogs will instinctively chase anything that moves past them very fast, whether animate or inanimate. Most then stop once they reach the target, although a few may then follow through with the next steps such as grab or even kill. In some breeds the chase instinct is particularly strong, especially herding breeds and sight hounds. They have been selectively bred to obtain a great deal of natural reward from chasing and will prefer to chase than do almost anything else. This can be problematic if directed at livestock, other pet animals or potentially dangerous targets such as cars.

Chase behaviour can be brought under control by teaching the puppy to respond to basic commands around structured chase games with balls or Frisbees. This not only enables the owner to control or interrupt chase behaviour, but also directs the puppy's focus on to chasing toys rather than other less suitable things. The puppy can initially be taught to perform a task for each throw of the toy, e.g. a 'sit'. He can then be taught to bring it back and gradually taught not to chase a thrown item until directed. This is best taught at training classes. It is best to avoid situations in which the puppy may be triggered to chase until he is old enough to start learning these commands to avoid the habit being established or increasing the reward the puppy gets from chasing unsuitable triggers.

Tug

It is sometimes suggested dogs should not be allowed to play tug with people, especially by dominance theorists who see it as a challenge for 'alpha'. Tug is part of the 'dissection' aspect of the hunting drive. It is therefore normal and part of every dog's behaviour. There will therefore be no undesirable consequences from playing tug freely and allowing the puppy to initiate and win the game in the vast majority of cases.

Tug toys for puppies need to have 'give' in them to avoid excessive pressure on the puppy's teeth. Examples include rubber tug toys or toys attached to some form of shock cord or bungee cord. Let the puppy actively pull whilst the person simply holds still, to ensure excessive pressure is not applied. Never forcibly remove the tug toy to end the game or remove the item from him. If the toy needs to be removed, manage in the same way as stealing (see Box 10.15).

If a dog has started to show signs of being aggressive over toys or to challenge the owner in certain circumstances it may be advisable to suspend tug games until the situation has been evaluated by an accredited behaviourist. In most cases playing tug will not be relevant to either development or correction of the behaviour. However, as the decision to use aggression is in part determined by the puppy's or dog's perception of whether he can win, often or always winning in a game of tug may very occasionally influence the puppy's perception he can do so.

Play signals

Some owners enjoy playing rough and tumble games with their dogs. This is fine. However, if they play this game with their owner there is a risk they may also try and do so with other people, who may not be so keen. This can be prevented by using a 'play' and 'stop' signal for this type of game. The signal can be verbal or physical, such as crossing the arms over the chest, but must be something people do not commonly do in everyday life or the puppy may interpret it as a sign to play at the wrong time. It is taught by routinely giving the signal before starting the game and refusing to play the game if initiated by the dog without it. The 'stop' signal is given at the end after which the owner refuses to play in this way anymore and redirects the puppy to play something else.

Manners

Dogs that have basic manners are far more pleasant to live with and are far less likely to develop problem behaviour. There are many ways to kindly teach manners, without the need to resort to dominance rituals, intimidation or punishment.

Saying please

Teaching a puppy to 'say please' simply refers to asking him to perform a task for the things he wants in life, typically a 'sit' but this can be modified according to the puppy. Doing so teaches the puppy he cannot simply take or demand things: he must ask instead. This has a far greater impact than just the act of asking the puppy to sit for a meal or for attention, in the same way as asking a child to 'say please' does. It also gently teaches him that these things are ultimately under his owner's control and so, whilst his owner will never harm or frighten him, the puppy does have to follow his owner's requests for calm and polite behaviour.

Teaching the puppy to ask instead of take also helps him to learn how to control his own behaviour. Young dogs often have too much energy and so may act impulsively: this is normal. However, it is not acceptable behaviour in an adult dog. Teaching the puppy to perform a calm task for things of value helps him learn how to exert self-control when he needs to.

This principle does not suggest excessive control of puppies. It does not limit their access to attention, food, the sofa or anything else they would like and their owner is happy for them to have. It also avoids using fear or intimidation if the puppy fails to ask nicely. It is not about trying to assert seniority or control. It is just teaching the puppy to show some self-control and consideration.

Training can be started as soon as the puppy knows what 'sit' means. In the early stages the puppy can be asked to 'sit' when he wants something so he understands what is required. Once the programme is started it is important to be consistent. If the task is not asked for consistently it will not be as effective. Young puppies are normally very compliant with this and if started early it is normally a habit by the time they reach puberty. However, if the puppy will not perform the required task then all that happens is he does not get what he wants until he has done so, just as a child does not get sweets if he does not say 'please'. Over time, doing so will often become a habit and so the prompt is no longer required. However, it can still be given if and when necessary. Never ignore a puppy's attempt to interact without first having asked him to 'sit' so he knows what is expected. Examples of what the puppy should be asked to sit for and how to do this are shown in Box 10.16.

Preventing aggression around food

Some dogs can become possessive around food. Traditionally dominance theorists often suggested that this was prevented by repeatedly taking the puppy's food away to teach him he is only allowed to have food if the owner says so. However, it is now recognized that doing so can increase rather than prevent food aggression by teaching the dog to expect it to be taken away.

Puppies can learn not to be concerned if people approach their food by teaching them this is a sign that more food is coming rather than the food being under threat. How to do so is summarized in Box 10.17. If a puppy or dog does start to show aggression around food the client should be referred to an accredited behaviourist as soon as possible (see Chapter 15).

Jumping up

Jumping up is normal dog behaviour. Dogs greet and communicate with each other at eye level. Large dogs will lower their head to get 'nose to nose' with smaller dogs. Small dogs and puppies will jump up on their hind legs to reach the face of larger or adult dogs. However, whilst it may be an

---

Box 10.16. Things puppies should be asked to 'say please' for.

- Having his lead on.
- Opening a door when he has asked to go out.
- Being allowed on to beds or sofas.
- When putting his food bowl down.
- Games.
- Attention.
- A new toy.
- A ball being thrown.

---

endearing habit in a puppy, jumping can be unpleasant or even dangerous in an adult and so should be discouraged. How to do so is summarized in Box 10.18.

Play biting

Dogs naturally use their mouths for exploration, manipulation and during play. Young puppies also learn how to control the pressure of their bite using their mouth on other dogs. Play biting, or 'mouthing', is therefore a normal and necessary part of social and physical development.

Using the mouth for exploration and manipulation is at its height during early development and most puppies will grow out of doing so other than in play. However, some may not, especially if they have learned that it is a reliable way to get attention from people, and some puppies may learn to use their mouth to manipulate others such as holding an owner's hand when they try to groom the puppy. In an older dog this can be painful and cause injuries, even if it is not true aggression. Therefore,

whilst mouthing should not be punished it should be controlled. How to do so is outlined in Box 10.19.

Whilst puppies should be taught not to mouth on people, they should be allowed to play bite with other dogs. This is normal social behaviour and prevention can interfere with development. It is also how the puppy learns to control his jaw and how much pressure he uses when he bites. How to manage and supervise play is discussed further in Chapters 5 and 11.

Children

Children and puppies are perfect playmates. Children have the energy to keep up with puppies and puppies teach children about responsibility, empathy and compassion. Both can teach the other to control impulsive behaviour. However, it is important that all interactions between puppies and children are guided and supervised.

Children can be involved with training from a very young age. Adults can command or elicit behaviours

---

Box 10.17. Teaching a puppy not to be worried by people approaching his food.

- The client should dish up 75% of the puppy's food ration.
- The puppy should be asked to sit whilst the bowl is put on the floor.
- The client should avoid taking the puppy's food away once he has started eating, unless in an emergency.
- As he is eating the client should approach him and drop one-third of the remainder in his bowl using a spoon, then walk away.

- This should be repeated with the remaining two portions.
- Once he knows the 'leave' command he can be asked to leave as they add the extra food.
- The client can also walk past the puppy as he is eating a high value food item such as a chew and drop a few treats on the floor by him, then walk away. Repeat regularly.
- How to remove things in an emergency is discussed in Box 10.15.

Box 10.18. Teaching a puppy not to jump up.

- Puppies should be greeted at their own level if possible. This will form a habit of having four paws on the ground whenever they greet.
- If a puppy jumps up to greet he should be asked to sit. Where possible the client should then get down to his level to greet him when he does so. People that find it hard to crouch down may find this easier if they always greet when sitting on a chair.

- If the puppy will not obey he should be ignored for about 10 sec then the 'sit' request repeated. If he persists use a 'time out' (see later in this chapter).
- The puppy should not be pushed down or shouted at as he may interpret this as a game or giving attention.
- All visitors should follow these principles. It may be wise to exclude the puppy until visitors are in and seated otherwise jumping up may be inadvertently rewarded whilst the owner is distracted.

---

and even toddlers can be the one to toss the treat or place the food bowl on the floor. Older children can give commands and reward with supervision and often quickly become enthusiastic about teaching tricks.

As much as the children need to teach the puppy how to behave they also have to learn how to behave around the puppy and respect the puppy's needs. This can be encouraged by teaching the child how to read signs that the puppy is unhappy as well as signs he is being playful. They will then know when to leave him alone.

It is absolutely essential that the puppy has the opportunity to get away from children once he has had enough. Provide an escape, such as a crate, to which the puppy always has access, and make it a golden rule that neither resident nor visiting children touch him when he is in there. Also teach children never to wake the puppy up wherever he is sleeping. This prevents the likelihood he may become worried around them and so feel the need to use threat to ask them to go away. It also helps make clear to the child that he has his own needs and feelings that must be respected.

Corrections

All puppies will sometimes show undesirable behaviour as part of growing up. It should be viewed as an opportunity to mould the puppy's behaviour into something more desirable. Using positive training methods does not mean allowing the puppy to do whatever he wants or to get into bad habits.

Always start by either redirecting the unwanted behaviour or commanding the puppy to do something else. For example, mouthing can be redirected on to a toy or jumping up can be prevented by asking the puppy to 'sit' to be greeted. If this does not work

and all of the puppy's needs have been met the puppy can then be given a consequence for his refusal to do so in the form of a negative punishment, i.e. by taking away something the puppy wants.

Ignore the behaviour

The usual process for training a puppy is to use food or a toy to 'lure' the puppy to perform a behaviour and then reward him for doing so. As the puppy starts to work out that performing the lured behaviour results in food he will start to do it more often. It can then be paired with a word and once the puppy has learned the word it can be used to ask the puppy to perform the behaviour without the need for the lure. In this situation the negative punishment is to withhold the reward, i.e. if the puppy does not go into the lured position, or perform the behaviour in response to the word once he knows it, then he will not receive the reward.

If rewards are withheld puppies often naturally try different ways to get them. This is referred to as 'trial and error'. In this situation the unwanted behaviours are ignored until the wanted behaviour occurs and is rewarded. Although it is often thought this is letting the puppy get away with 'naughty' behaviour it is in fact another example of negative punishment, i.e. the puppy is not being given the reward that he wants whilst performing unwanted behaviour. When he then tries something else more desirable, which he invariably will, he then gets the reward.

Ignore the puppy

If a puppy is performing behaviours that it is impossible to ignore and will not stop when given an alternative command or redirected on to something else, it can be very effective to then ignore the puppy. This is quite different to just ignoring behaviour as it involves turning away from, avoiding looking at, not speaking to and not acknowledging the puppy at all.

Puppies must never be ignored without first being told what to do. It is something that bothers the puppy quite a lot and he will not understand if what he sees as perfectly normal behaviour such as jumping up results in social exclusion. However, if the client has tried to redirect the behaviour and the puppy will not obey then they can ignore him until the unwanted behaviour stops. They can then repeat the alternative command and reward the good behaviour when it occurs.

Once started it is important the client sees the punishment though. If they relent after a moment or two they will have actually made the behaviour worse by teaching the puppy he has to persist with the unwanted behaviour for a while before he gets want he wants, just like the child that learns he has to ask for sweets five times before his mother will give in. It is also important that the client is consistent. If they only withhold the reward some of the time the puppy will feel it is always worth trying to see if he can get his own way.

Time out

In situations where it is impossible to ignore the puppy it may be necessary to use a 'time out'.

This involves leaving the puppy alone for just a couple of minutes. How to impose the time out is summarized in Box 10.20. 'Time out' should not be used for puppies that suffer with separation issues. Owners also need to ensure their puppy knows the difference between exclusion as a consequence and exclusion for management, e.g. when a caller arrives. This can be achieved by speaking to the puppy in a jolly way or leaving him with a toy or treat when excluding him from the latter.

Puppies should never be subjected to positive punishment or, by association, negative reward. As discussed in Chapter 7 incorrect use of positive punishments can cause a number of different problems, including a breakdown in puppy–owner relationship, fear, on-going anxiety and pre-emptive defensive aggression. Puppy behaviour can always be managed using positive reward and negative punishments. If the owner or their current trainer/behaviourist does not know how to do so they can be referred to someone trained in these methods (see Chapter 15).

Acceptance of Handling

Puppies can be taught from a young age to accept being handled in ways that will be necessary as he grows up by performing the tasks outlined in Table 42 regularly in a calm and positive way. Ideally these will be performed a few at a time over a number of sessions. Give treats, fuss or toys during or after doing so. Observe the puppy's body language and stop if

---

Box 10.20. Using a 'time out'.

- The most effective way to give a 'time out' is to leave the room and close the door. This is preferable because it can be performed without giving the puppy the inevitable attention that accompanies taking him out of the room. It also avoids the need to chase, corner or drag the puppy, which risk becoming a game or causing pain or fear. In most cases only the person the unwanted behaviour is being directed at needs to leave as they are the person the puppy wants at that time.
- If there is a reason the puppy is unable to be left where he is, he can be calmly led out of the room and put behind a door. Ensure he is not spoken to or looked at whilst doing so. Avoid excess force or handling he may find distressing. Pick him up, but do not cuddle, if this helps. A house line (a long line with no loop, which is left on the puppy when

in company) may help ensure the puppy can be caught without it becoming a game of chase.
- The puppy's bed, den or crate should not be used for 'time out'.
- It is essential the 'time out' is given immediately and every time the behaviour occurs. Delays mean the puppy may link the 'time out' to the wrong thing or become confused. Inconsistency will make the puppy feel it is worth at least trying to get his own way.
- The time out should be for 30 s for very young puppies, rising to 2 min for older ones.
- Once the puppy is let back in the punishment is over. The owner should then direct the puppy onto something suitable.
- The time out may need to be repeated a few times before the puppy works out what it is for via 'trial and error'.

Table 42. Teaching a puppy to feel comfortable being handled.

Task	Description
Name body parts	Touch various parts of the body, such as the ear, tail or foot. Say their name and give the puppy a treat.
Open mouth	Open the puppy's mouth and pop a treat in.
Look in and sniff ears	Lift the ear flap and sniff the puppy's ears. Gently massage the ear base and give a treat.
Massage scruff	Massage the scruff and give the puppy a treat.
Squeeze toes	Pick up the foot and gently squeeze each toe as if clipping claws and give a treat.
Touch under tummy	Rub the puppy under the tummy as he is standing up and give a treat.
Lift up tail	Lift up the puppies tail and look underneath and give a treat.
Groom	Start to gently brush and comb the puppy whilst giving treats.
Teeth	Put some dog toothpaste on a finger and rub it over your puppy's teeth.

the puppy looks fearful or threatening. In this case refer the client to an accredited behaviourist.

Collars and leads

Puppies need to learn to accept wearing a collar and lead. These are not harmful but some puppies may take a while to get used to them. Use a soft flat collar and make sure it is checked regularly and adjusted or replaced as the puppy grows. Start by putting the collar on during meals or periods of play to distract the puppy from it. Once the puppy happily accepts the collar, start to attach a trailing lead.

The aim will be to teach the puppy to walk on the lead without pulling and to use commands to control him. However, there may be times when someone restrains him by the lead or takes hold of his collar to control behaviour, either inadvertently or out of necessity if he will not obey a command. Therefore it helps to teach the puppy not to be worried by this. Occasionally take hold of the puppy's collar and give him a treat. There is no need to apply pressure or hold firmly to get the desired effect – simply teach the puppy that having his collar held is of no concern. Also walk him using the loose lead and if he pulls call him back to you in a jolly way. This teaches him that a tight lead is not a signal of danger without the risk of rewarding him for pulling.

Puppy Training

Puppies can start training as soon as they get home. The earlier they learn commands the more reliably they will obey them as they get older. It is also possible to manipulate natural puppy behaviours to help with training. The principles of training are discussed in Chapter 7. How to train key basic commands is discussed in Appendix 6. Puppies have very short attention spans, so training sessions should be no more than 2–3 min each and performed regularly throughout the day. If the puppy is not focusing, then abandon the session and try again later.

Even where an owner is a competent trainer there is still a great deal of value in taking puppies to puppy classes. These not only help with training but also provide valuable socialization to strangers and other puppies. Owners must take great care when choosing the class to which to take their puppy. This is the most critical period of the puppy's life and so it is essential they only attend good quality professionally run classes based on up to date understanding of dog training and behaviour. The emphasis needs to be on puppies learning to be well behaved rather than obedient, i.e. that they choose good behaviour because it gets them the best outcome rather than constantly having to be told what to do. Guidelines for running classes in the practice are discussed in Chapter 11. How to choose a trainer or puppy adviser is discussed in Chapter 15.

Juvenile Behaviour

Puppies undergo a further period of intense development around puberty, which needs to be carefully managed. Key changes likely to occur are as follows.

Growth

As puppies physically grow they have more energy and need less sleep. However, although they are the size of an adult dog, they still have the enthusiasm, curiosity and tendency to seek activity that a puppy does. This can be trying for owners, especially with larger breeds, and is commonly a time for relinquishment.

Management relies on using the same principles as for younger puppies but increasing the quantity and complexity of exercise and stimulation offered. Tips for fulfilling the older puppies' needs are summarized in Box 10.21.

Puberty

As the puppy reaches puberty circulating sex hormones start to rise. Just as in humans this may result in changes in behaviour as the puppy adjusts to their effects on emotions and behaviour. Levels may also fluctuate at first leading to day-to-day variations in behaviour. Typical changes are as follows.

Dispersal

Many puppies start to be more willing to move further away from the owner. This is linked to normal dispersal behaviour at puberty. This can be managed through increased recall training or transient use of a long line if needed.

Sexual behaviour

The puppy may start to show interest in dogs of the opposite sex or competition to dogs of the same sex, especially around the first season in females. The puppy may also start to frequently mount other dogs or inanimate objects, especially males. Dogs that do so excessively and whose arousal does not pass may be good candidates for neutering (also see Chapter 7).

Boundary testing

Some puppies may try to test the boundaries for acceptable behaviour or human reactions to low-level threat when they get to puberty as many teenage humans would. This may be seen as refusal to obey commands, use of low-level aggression if given a command, or threat to keep possession of items or control others' behaviour. At this stage the puppy's body language is often a mixture of threat and appeasing or play, lacking the true menace of an adult.

Boundary testing can be prevented from becoming a long-term problem by calmly continuing with the training discussed above. Wilfulness can be stopped by introducing higher value treats, increasing frequency of practice sessions and negative punishment.

Threats should not be punished as this is just as likely to lead to an escalation as it is for the puppy to back down. Most puppies respond very well to a calm but firm alternative command at this time, such as asking him to 'sit' or calling him back to

---

Box 10.21. Occupying an older puppy.

- Ensure the puppy has been taught a recall command to enable off-lead exercise. If his recall breaks down use of lunge lines/long flat leads or exercise paddocks enable exercise levels to be maintained.
- He should be given free access to suitable toys that are rotated to maintain interest. Their scent can be changed before giving back to increase their interest.
- The puppy can be taught 'fetch', which can then be played on walks or in the garden.
- Dog walkers can be used where the owner cannot provide enough exercise.
- Periods should be allocated for play throughout the day. This creates a habit that reduces mischief at other times and ensures it is not overlooked.
- All meals can be fed in treat balls, Kongs or other toys. Scatter-feeding in the garden in dry weather also helps.

- The puppy can be taken to dog sports or classes suited to his age.
- Some puppies enjoy a badger box made from a large cardboard box that is sealed with tape and has any staples removed. A hole is made in one corner and it is filled with screwed up newspaper, treats and toys. The puppy is allowed to get in and remove the items.
- Some puppies enjoy Russian doll boxes: cardboard boxes (after any staples have been removed) are layered inside each other with a treat or toy at each layer. The puppy is allowed to dismember it.
- Toilet roll tubes and empty bottles can be filled with treats and sealed and the puppy allowed to dismember them.

NB All toys designed to be ripped up can only be given under supervision and to those puppies that do not swallow the pieces from things he has chewed up.

---

you and then rewarding him. If this does not work or the puppy is using higher level or more intense threat the owner should withdraw and be referred to an accredited behaviourist.

Second fear period

It is common for puppies to go through a period of heightened sensitivity or to become fearful of things that did not used to concern them around the time of puberty. It is not fully understood why some dogs do this, but it is possible there is a genetic predisposition to it. Most dogs normally pass through this phase as they mature, as long as it is not aggravated or reinforced in some way.

Owners should neither pay extra attention to or ignore the puppy if he behaves fearfully. They should stay calm and treat the puppy in the same way they always do. The puppy should be allowed to withdraw to a place where he feels safe to prevent the unpleasant sensations of fear intensifying his perception that the trigger is unpleasant. The client must never show anger to, punish or force the puppy to face the trigger. The owner can try interacting with the trigger him or herself to show that it is interesting and safe. The puppy can also be exposed to the trigger in a diluted form and played with or given treats to link the trigger to positive emotions (see above). If the puppy is still showing fear the client should be referred to an accredited behaviourist.

Getting Professional Help

Even where the owner has followed all the guidelines there may still be times where the puppy's behaviour becomes worrying or dangerous. There will also be times where owners have perhaps made mistakes or been given poor advice, or where puppies have been rehomed or rescued. Where there is any sign things are going wrong the help of an accredited behaviourist should be sought as a matter of urgency. The rate of success for correcting problem behaviour reduces dramatically the longer it is allowed to continue. This is particularly true with puppies who are still developing and learning about their world and whose neural pathways are rapidly developing and becoming established. Early intervention therefore gives the greatest chance of success. How to choose whose advice to seek is discussed in Chapter 15.

Additional Resources

Helen Zulch and Daniel Mills (2012) *Life Skills for Puppies: Laying the foundation for a loving, lasting relationship.* Veloce Publishing Ltd, Dorchester, UK.
Gwenn Bailey (2008) *The Perfect Puppy.* Hamlyn, London.

Resources to teach children to behave safely around dogs

The Kennel Club – Safe and Sound Scheme. Available at: http:// www.safetyarounddogs.org.uk

11 Running Puppy Socialization Classes

Aims

Many practices offer puppy socialization classes, often referred to as 'puppy parties'. They are typically but not exclusively led by veterinary nurses or technicians. The benefits of running such classes may include bonding the client to the practice, promoting a positive practice image and improving the likely behaviour of the adult dog in practice. For practices that charge they can also provide an income stream. Whatever the intention it is critical that the staff running these classes are properly trained and that the aims of each session are carefully thought through. Puppy classes can be very useful for ensuring proper development and preventing problem behaviour later in life. However, if run poorly they can do more harm than good at this critical time in the puppy's life, which may be hard to undo at a later stage. Therefore, as with the education of children, only those that have the required expertise and experience should be entrusted with the task of doing so.

The key stages of puppy development are discussed in Chapter 2. Understanding canine communication, and being able to identify normal play or signs of worry or threat is discussed in Chapter 5. Training and puppy behaviour management are discussed in Chapter 10. It is important to read and fully understand all these chapters before assisting at puppy classes. It is also important to develop practical knowledge and skills by either acting as an assistant under supervision of a more experienced member of staff or, if starting classes for the first time in the practice, by attending other classes in the area for supervised hands-on experience. It may also help to ask an accredited behaviourist, trainer or veterinary nurse or technician experienced in puppy rearing to help run the first few classes to help with teething problems or any issues.

The key aims of puppy socialization classes are summarized in Table 43.

Class Format

Fixed or rolling admission

The frequency and duration of classes and protocol for accepting new puppies will be in part dictated by the number of puppies the practice sees and staff availability. Ideally classes will be held at least weekly to ensure puppies have the opportunity to attend at the right stage of development. The optimum number of sessions each puppy should attend is four to ensure regular socialization and time to cover all the subject areas without cramming. Duration needs to take into account that very young puppies have a poor attention span and need frequent periods of rest, which they may be reluctant to take when surrounded by other puppies and people. They therefore should not be longer than 1 h. Classes are often held in the evening when the practice is quiet and the business of the day concluded. However, this requires a greater commitment by practice staff and may make some owner's reluctant to attend, especially when it is dark in the evenings. If facilities and timetabling allow, mid-afternoon sessions may therefore be more practical and popular in some cases.

Classes can be run as a fixed course or on a roll-on, roll-off basis. A fixed course of classes enables content to be structured to avoid repetition. It also enables puppies to make friends, which can help shy puppies relax. However, it can result in long delays before new puppies can start. Some may even miss out altogether if they are already old enough for training classes by the time the next course starts. Rolling classes involve two to four sessions repeated on a continuous cycle. Puppies can join as soon as they are ready and leave once they have attended all four sessions, or when they are ready for training classes. This prevents any delay in starting classes and increases the number of other puppies and people each puppy will meet as puppies leave and new ones join.

Table 43. Key aims of puppy socialization classes.

Aim	Discussion
Socialization	Classes provide the opportunity for puppies to meet different types of people and other dogs in a structured way that ensures these experiences are positive. They also enable development of dog–dog social skills.
Habituation	Classes provide the opportunity for puppies to experience a wide range of stimuli in a structured way to ensure the experiences are positive. They also enable puppies to have repeated pleasant visits to the practice to provide protection against developing future fear of doing so.
Education of owner	Classes can provide invaluable information and practical guidance for first-time owners or those whose knowledge may be out of date.
Early training	Guidance can be given in how to teach key basic commands that enable early management and prevention of problem behaviour.
Bonding to the practice	Clients that have a positive experience at puppy classes are much more likely to continue to use the practice as the puppy grows up.
Identifying puppies that need extra help	Early intervention provides the best prognosis for puppies showing early problem behaviour or clients that need extra support. Classes enable these to be identified.

Class size

Class sizes need to be carefully controlled. If classes are too small they do not offer optimal socialization but if they are too large they may be intimidating for smaller or shy puppies. Optimum size is between four and eight, depending on the size and character of the puppies and the level of experience of those running it. Class size will also depend on the number and ability of staff available. Aim for a ratio of one assistant to every two to three puppies.

Age of admission

The age at which puppies can start classes will need to be decided by the veterinary team. A puppy's sensitivity to accepting new things without concern starts to wane from about 8 weeks. The greatest behavioural advantage is therefore achieved if puppies join as soon as they come to live with their new owner. However, this has to be balanced against protection from disease. The considerations when doing so are summarized in Table 44. It must be remembered that both disease and poor socialization and habituation carry equal risk of long-term harm or loss of life (see box in Introduction).

The age at which puppies should stop attending is determined by a combination of having attended all the sessions, being ready to move on to puppy training classes and the individual size and behaviour of the puppy. In larger practices classes can be continued by running concurrent groups for young, small or quiet puppies and larger, older and more boisterous puppies.

Who should attend

Only healthy puppies should attend. If there is any sign of illness or injury the puppy should not be allowed to come to avoid disease transmission or the association of pain with puppy play or the practice. Owners can still be encouraged to attend and be given guidance on training and socialization that can be performed away from classes.

Ideally all of a puppy's family will attend classes to ensure they are all aware of the key messages each class covers. However, if the puppy belongs to a large family this may be overwhelming for the other puppies. It is therefore wise to restrict numbers to two or three people per puppy per week. It is also important that any children attending can be relied on to do as asked. Practice staff should have no compunction about not permitting unruly children to attend and asking them to leave if they misbehave. It is better to exclude children under 5 as they require too much supervision and are not yet able to follow direction reliably. For some puppies this will be their first experience with children and so it must be a positive one. Children must be supervised by parents throughout the class and supported whilst learning how to handle the puppies. It can also help to provide things for children

Table 44. Matters for consideration when choosing the starting age for puppy socialization classes.

Consideration	Discussion
Disease risk in the practice	The risk of exposure to contagious diseases. This can be controlled through use of specialist disinfectants and practice expertise in preventing disease transmission. Specific protocols need to be drawn up to ensure these are followed.
Vaccination protocols	The protection offered at first and second vaccination by the practice vaccination protocol.
Sensitive periods	Sensitive periods for socialization and habituation peak at 8 weeks and then taper until approximately 13 weeks at which they close. The more time the puppy can spend in structured socialization and habituation training before the sensitive period ends, the less risk there is of problem behaviour in later life. Variations in sensitive periods between breeds also need to be considered.
Source of puppy	Where the puppy came from will affect the likelihood he is incubating a disease that could be passed on to others. Equally there is a need to actively compensate for early deprivation in outdoor or puppy-farmed individuals.

to do, such as colouring books or puppy-proof toys, in case they get bored or fractious.

Invitations

Paper invitations can be given at the first puppy vaccination to ensure all puppy owners are made aware of class availability. Booking can be made at reception, online or by ringing the practice to keep numbers within target.

Costs

Whether to charge for attendance is a practice decision. Many practices are happy to bear the cost of classes as part of their service to their clients and for the longer term benefits derived. They also often find that the costs are covered by sales on the night. Alternatively it may be possible to obtain sponsorship from puppy-related product or service providers.

There is also an argument for making a nominal charge. This may deter some clients from booking but tends to increase actual attendance once a booking has been made and would add value to the class in the eyes of many clients. Giving free gifts, such as a good quality book or puppy toy, or practice vouchers to the value of the fee paid may reduce concerns about costs and make clients feel they are getting value for money.

Environment and Equipment

The location for the classes needs to be safe and secure. It must be entirely enclosed to prevent escapees and have either a permanent or temporary double-door system or suitable locks to prevent doors being unexpectedly opened. It is important that the room layout enables all the puppies to be supervised at all times by assistants.

All surfaces must be washable and cleaned with a suitable disinfectant effective against all communicable diseases before puppies are admitted. The room should be checked for potential hazards and these removed or made inaccessible.

Chairs are best arranged in small groups. Avoid one large group or rows of chairs. Make sure there is space between the chairs so shy puppies can withdraw if they want to.

Use of temporary pens or barriers can help control where puppies can go and prevent access to areas that cannot be properly disinfected, e.g. soft furnishings. They can also be used to separate excitable puppies from others during quiet times. Changing the room layout each week provides novelty to keep interest and maximize the effect of habituation.

Providing novel objects can help puppies learn about their world and to cope with new things. Socialization to people can be enhanced by providing different types of clothing such as wigs, false beards, reflective sunglasses, motorcycle helmets, umbrellas, walking sticks, fluorescent jackets, rucksacks and hats for people to dress up in. Suitable washable interactive and solitary play toys can be made available and rotated weekly to provide stimulation and to give clients inspiration for how to occupy their puppy at home. Clients can be encouraged to bring their own treats or their puppy's kibble but there will be times when something more motivating is required. Such treats need to be small, low calorie whilst desirable and unlikely to trigger digestive upset in young puppies.

Background noise tapes can introduce novel sounds but care must be taken not to startle the more sensitive puppies. Start very quietly and gradually increase to a comfortable background level as long as none of the puppies seems fearful. Owners can be encouraged to conduct this type of training at home to continue habituation and enable the sounds to be played at a louder level suited to the individual puppy's needs. This is particularly important for sound-sensitive breeds such as herding breeds.

Provide access to an outdoor area puppies can be taken to if they show signs of wanting to eliminate. Owners should be encouraged to take their puppy there before the class starts. Encourage owners to bring their own portable drinking bowls to avoid cross-contamination.

Class Planning and Content

It is important to structure classes to ensure all subject matter and experiences are covered and to promote a professional image. The act of planning also helps focus the mind on how sessions should be run. Suitable activities are as follows.

Client education

Classes offer an excellent opportunity to educate clients in all aspects of puppy care including health, husbandry and behaviour management. The behavioural subjects recommended for discussion are summarized in Box 11.1 and covered in more detail in Chapters 2, 4, 5 and 10. Spend a few minutes discussing the key points of three or four subjects each week, whilst the puppies are resting (see below). The information given can be supported with hand-outs or web resources, or by directing clients to suitable books.

Give each owner all the written resources at their first visit so these are available if needed prior to being discussed in subsequent classes.

Mock examinations

In-practice classes provide an opportunity to teach puppies to enjoy being examined and being in the practice. Take puppies individually into a consulting room with their owner. Allow the puppy to explore the room and to approach the staff member voluntarily. Once the puppy seems comfortable with the staff member place a few treats on the table and ask the owner to lift him on to it. Allow him to eat the treats. The staff member can then gently check all over whilst the owner gives treats. The puppy can also be lured on to cat-weighing scales using treats or a little suitable food paste. Monitor the puppy's body language throughout the mock examination to ensure this is a positive experience. Stop if the puppy seems concerned at any stage. If this occurs it may help to arrange for the puppy to visit the practice again during the day so he can be habituated to being there before examination is tried, and examinations can be allowed to proceed more slowly. If the puppy continues to show signs of stress advise the client to seek help from an accredited behaviourist.

Introductions to strangers and other puppies

Providing opportunities to meet new people and other puppies is one of the key aims of the puppy socialization class. However, this needs to managed according to each puppy's individual temperament to avoid causing rather than preventing problems.

Box 11.1. Behaviour subjects to discuss during puppy socialization classes.

- Canine drives, needs and social behaviour, including discussion of why dominance theories are outdated.
- Understanding body language.
- Socialization and habituation.
- Play and stimulation.
- Teaching children how to behave around puppies.
- Toilet training.

- Manners.
- Basic training and choosing a trainer.
- Crates and playpens.
- Jumping up.
- Mouthing.
- Chewing.
- Stealing.
- Juvenile behaviour and puberty.

Greeting to people

It is essential to read and fully understand Chapter 5 before supervising interactions with strangers. Introductions should be made to one new person at a time. Avoid 'round robin' or pass the puppy sessions. Ideally each puppy will be allowed to initially meet new people without the other person's puppy being there, although this will depend on whether there is someone else the other person's puppy knows to look after him whilst doing so. Ask the puppy owner and new person to sit on the floor, if they are able, away from the rest of the group. Release the puppy and allow him to approach the stranger rather than the person approaching him or having the puppy passed to him. The stranger should not lure the puppy to them but can reward him with some treats or play if he chooses to approach. They can then greet the puppy by stroking under the chin or on the bib. They should then intermittently stop fussing to see if the puppy invites them to carry on. Most will but the person should not press the puppy if he is not keen.

Matching puppies for interaction

Interaction with other puppies is best performed in groups of three. This reduces the pressure on each individual puppy and makes it easier for a shy or reticent puppy to withdraw whilst keeping the group small enough for each individual puppy's behaviour to be monitored. Avoid free play in large groups.

The puppies need to be matched according to size, age, physical strength, styles of play, confidence and individual character. Table 45 highlights the key considerations when choosing which puppies to place together. Ensure that large or overly confident puppies are not placed with small or shy puppies. Be aware of the types of games breeds play and aim to balance these. For example, German shepherds tend to bowl other dogs over and bull breeds can be mouthy. They therefore are not suited to gentler breeds such as collies or lap dogs that prefer to chase and have minimal contact. The skills needed to match puppies will be learned during practical sessions with a more experienced nurse or technician, or an accredited trainer or behaviourist as discussed above. If there are no suitable matches or you are not confident of being able to identify suitable play partners it is better to skip play sessions than permit play that may lead to problem behaviour.

If two puppies are attending together (e.g. siblings), arrange for them to play separately with other puppies to give them the opportunity to learn how to interact with unfamiliar dogs. Groups of puppies can be separated by directing them into separate consulting rooms, or using screens or a circle of chairs. Each group must be supervised.

Interacting with other puppies

It is essential to read and fully understand Chapter 5 and to develop practical experience as discussed above before being in sole charge of supervising interactions between puppies.

Interaction between the puppies must be carefully controlled to ensure bullies are not encouraged and to prevent worried puppies becoming more so or learning to use aggression to control other dogs. This may the first time some puppies have met other dogs,

Table 45. Factors to consider when evaluating differences in individual puppy temperament.

Factor	Discussion
Age	Although the range of ages will be numerically small it will span a period of rapid development. Each puppy's stage on that process therefore needs to be considered.
Size and physical strength	Larger puppies may inadvertently worry smaller puppies or cause distress simply due to variations in size. Breeds of the same size may also vary in physical strength or strength of bite. Gentle sensitive breeds should not be paired with stronger powerful breeds even if they match in size.
Breed	Breeds enter fear periods at different ages and vary in sociability to other dogs and style of play.
Confidence	A strong pushy puppy may intimidate a shyer less confident individual, aggravating their behaviour.
Length of ownership	The longer the puppy has been with their current owner, the more relaxed and confident the puppy is likely to be.
Source	Consider how much the puppy has been socialized and habituated prior to acquisition.
Individual temperament	Every puppy is an individual and so must be observed to assess individual traits

other than their dam and siblings. It is therefore critical this is a positive experience.

Allow the puppies to approach and greet each other and monitor body language to ensure they are all comfortable and keen to interact with each other. Watch for normal social greeting and play signals (see Fig. 8). Ensure any puppy can withdraw at any time and separate in a calm and jolly way if any aspect of the play is unacceptable (see Chapter 5 and Boxes 11.2, 11.3). Aim to separate by calling or luring the puppies away. If this is not effective gently pick up the puppies and walk them away, then direct them on to something else fun, e.g. a tuggy toy. If you are unsure whether or not to break up the session, separate the puppies and then release the least confident. If he returns to play this suggests he did not find it worrying. End play sessions after about 3–4 min. They can be repeated throughout the class. Give owners a running commentary during play so they learn what to look for when supervising puppy play. This is a huge opportunity for owners to learn how to read their dog and know when to allow and when to interrupt play. If you are not confident at being able to manage play then seek guidance from an accredited behaviourist or attend other parties or training classes to develop your skills.

Supervision and rotation

If there are insufficient staff to supervise each group of puppies then stagger play sessions and give other attendees something to do, e.g. browse stock, read posters and literature or play one to one with their own puppy away from the others.

Rotate the person and puppy each puppy interacts with every week, as long as there enough suitable matches. If this is not possible ask owners to use the clothing items above to make themselves appear different.

Recalls and passing by

Each owner should intermittently call their puppies back during free interaction and reward them for doing so. This will start to teach the puppy to come away from distractions. The owner may need to be quite animated to encourage their puppy to come back to them rather than continue the game. If this does not work the owner can also try a food lure or a squeaky ball to gain the puppy's attention. If he still ignores the recall the owner should calmly interrupt play and remove the puppy from the play area. The client may then need additional help from an accredited trainer to help with this. It is also important that puppies learn to greet another dog then focus back on to the owners or walk on so they learn they cannot always stop and play. Incorporate brief periods of walking the puppies on lead during the class. Give plenty of space between puppies and watch for any that seem worried. Confident puppies can be allowed to approach each other, sniff in greeting then be called away by their owner in a calm and jolly way after a few seconds. The owner should reward the puppy for coming with fuss or a treat, depending what the puppy responds best to. If the puppy shows any signs of worry they should be allowed to withdraw and then exclude them from the activity. Refer the client to an accredited behaviourist.

Box 11.2. Monitoring puppy play (also see Chapter 5).

- Observe for play signals such as a play bow, pounce or turning in a 360° circle.
- Observe for equally matched play bouts. Puppies should take turns in who chases who and which is on their back during wrestling bouts. If one puppy is always on top, always pinning the other down or always chasing the other, interrupt the session.
- An element of mounting is common in play but where this is repeated or the puppy being mounted looks concerned, interrupt.
- Play normally stops and starts during which each puppy responds to the other's signals. If there are no natural gaps in play bouts separate the puppies

briefly and look for mutual play signals suggesting both want to start again.
- Body language should be relaxed throughout. Soft faces, bent legs, open mouths and relaxed sweeping tails all suggest relaxed play. If either puppy looks still, stiff or is showing signs of worry, separate and test whether both parties want to play again.
- Play is normally fairly quiet. If it becomes too noisy this suggests over excitement, fear or aggression and so needs to be interrupted.
- Stop play if either puppy is showing any sign of threat, strong appeasement or looks worried or tired. Stop play if one makes the other squeal.

Quiet periods

Teaching puppies to be calm in distracting situations is as important as teaching social skills. Doing so can easily be incorporated into classes such as when discussing the various aspects of canine behaviour discussed above or whilst other puppies are playing if there are not enough staff to supervise multiple small play sessions.

Puppies can be encouraged to sit quietly on their owner's lap or on a mat. Owners should be encouraged to bring suitable calming or food toys with them such as stuffed Kongs or puppy chews to settle the puppy at such times. Screens can be used to separate puppies if the sight of another puppy is causing excitement. If a puppy is getting particularly restless or noisy it may help if they are held by someone else providing they are confident to do so, or by the owner standing up and walking about. This might be an opportune time for the owner to browse the stock or take the puppy to the outside toileting area for a few minutes. Shy puppies can be moved to a side room with a baby gate across the door to help them observe from a safe distance. It is important not to resort to water pistols, bitter sprays, air canisters or any other aversive methods to silence noisy puppies. See Chapter 7 regarding the concerns associated with their use.

Guest speakers

Guest speakers can provide variety and specialist information on subjects with which staff are not comfortable. If offered by local trainers they can also lead in to on-going puppy services. See Chapter 15 regarding how to identify a suitable trainer or behaviourist to invite.

Basic training

Clients should be encouraged to take their puppy to basic training classes with a qualified trainer as soon as they are old enough. However, teaching the puppy to perform key behaviours on 'command' or 'cue' can be started at puppy socialization classes. The most important behaviours to teach early are summarized in Table 46. How to teach each of these is explained in Appendix 6. Only positive reward methods should be used. Puppies are very biddable at this age and respond very easily to lures and rewards. Use of dominance/pack leader or positive punishment methods can cause serious and at times irreversible damage and is a common cause of later euthanasia on behavioural grounds. The reasons for this and dangers of using these methods are discussed further in Chapters 4 and 7.

Sales

Clients often value the opportunity to purchase suitable products for their puppies under the guidance of a knowledgeable professional. Sales can also help cover the cost of parties where no charge is made, or clients can be given a voucher to redeem against purchases to encourage booking where a fee is charged.

Examples of the types of products to sell are summarized in Table 47. They must be selected carefully to ensure they are the best available as they will no doubt set the precedence for the types of products the client uses for the rest of their dog's life.

Table 46. Priority commands to teach at puppy socialization classes.

Behaviour	Reason for use
Sit	'Sit' is very easy to teach to most breeds. Once established it can be used to teach the puppy manners, to ask a puppy to be calm or asked for as an alternative behaviour that can then be rewarded if a puppy is doing something unwanted.
Stay	Enables the puppy's behaviour to be managed in a variety of situations such as when greeting people, opening doors or leaving the puppy alone for a few minutes.
Recall	Being able to call a puppy or dog back is essential for good manners, freedom and safety. Puppies are very receptive to coming when called at this age. This should be taken advantage of to teach a reliable recall early so this becomes a force of habit in later life.
Give and leave	Puppies commonly steal during their early months. How this is managed can make a huge difference to the dog's behaviour in later life. Teaching a puppy to happily leave or give up things enables this to be done without causing friction or making stealing an attention-seeking game.

Table 47. Products to sell and considerations for their selection.

Product group	Considerations
Toys	Toys need to be safe, durable and desirable. Puppies will require toys that both fulfil their natural drives, such as to rip things up and tug, and teach them to calm down. Calming toys involve those that are designed to be filled with food but require the dog to sit quietly to get it out such as Kongs and Traxx. Avoid chase toys at this stage, especially in herding breeds, to prevent this becoming too strong before the puppy is ready to be taught to do so in a controlled way.
Treats	Treats should be small and low calorie. They also need to be desirable to the puppy. It can help to have a few of each treat available to try so the owner can test which their puppy prefers.
Collar, leads, head collars and harnesses	Puppies are best initially familiarized to wearing soft neck collars with flat leads. There should not be any need to use head collars or harnesses to prevent pulling at this age, although some breeds are better suited to a flat rigid body harness. Avoid harnesses that tighten as the puppy pulls at this stage. Actively discourage owners from using check/choke or prong/pinch collars or slip leads. The concerns regarding their use are summarized in Chapter 7.
Books and training materials	Any books or other training or puppy advice resources offered should be carefully read to ensure the contents reflect the principles being taught during the classes.
Sound CDs	Sound CDs can enable owners to continue sound habituation at home, especially in sound-sensitive breeds. Read the instruction manual provided with the CD and provide practice instructions where this is inadequate or not present.

Homework

Give clients targets for socialization and training for the next week to ensure they are using the time between classes constructively. Provide socialization charts and reading material or resources, and a point of contact if they need further advice.

Puppies Showing Problem Behaviour

Always be on the lookout for early signs of problem behaviour. These may arise due to poor early handling or socialization with the breeder, inappropriate handling by the owner, a poor match between owner and puppy, genetics or any of the other influences over behaviour discussed in Chapter 2.

Shy puppies

Being able to identify and properly manage shy puppies is a critical skill for the veterinary nurse or technician when running puppy classes. How to identify body language that shows a puppy is worried is discussed in Chapter 5. Key signs of stress are also summarized in Box 11.3.

Ensure puppies that lack confidence or show signs of worry are not overwhelmed. It may help to allow shy puppies to initially watch from the safety of a consulting room separated from the main area by a baby gate. If their confidence grows they can then be allowed to interact with other quiet gentle puppies as discussed above.

If the puppy is showing signs of stress or defensive behaviour even in the refuge remove him from the class completely. Do not be tempted to try and address this puppy's problem behaviour in future classes or in house consultations. Refer the client and puppy to an accredited behaviourist (see Chapter 15). Ensure the owner knows how important it is to do so without delay if their puppy is to be given the best chance of overcoming this current level of fear. They must understand he will not 'grow out of it' and that this type of early fearfulness generally tends to get gradually worse and be harder to undo with every passing month. Early intervention is therefore critical.

Excitable, pushy or mismatched puppy/owner combinations

Puppies that are overly excitable, are very pushy or are a poor match for their owner's personality or circumstances also need early specialist help. These puppies are at risk of either being allowed to run riot or being subjected to punishments as their increasingly frustrated or exasperated owners try to bring their behaviour under control. The risks associated with doing so are discussed in Chapter 7. They should again be referred to an accredited behaviourist.

Box 11.3. Signs of stress.

- Licking lips or nose.
- Chomping (like chewing a toffee).
- Yawning.
- Puffing out cheeks.
- Hesitant, reluctant or watchful behaviour.
- Wet dog shake.
- Tail lowered/between legs.
- Ears flattened against head.
- Head lowered and tucked to cover neck.
- Cowering.
- Trembling.
- Drooling.
- Panting.
- Refusing treats.
- Whining or high-pitched anxious bark.
- Trying to hide or escape.
- Urinating without normal preliminary behaviour.
- Freezing.
- Growling or snarling.

12 Managing Behaviour in Ill Health

The potential behavioural effects of ill health are discussed in Chapter 2. In many cases correction of the health concern will resolve the problem behaviour. However, in some cases the illness may have a transient or long-term effect on behaviour, which needs to be managed.

Debilitating Illness, Convalescence and Palliative Care

Many illnesses affect a dog's ability to function normally, which will in turn affect their behaviour or emotional state. This applies equally whether the illness is transient or terminal. Steps need to be taken to manage these changes.

Aggression and fear

Dogs that are in pain often become fearful of the painful or injured part of the body being handled. In many cases this leads to withdrawal or strong appeasing behaviour. In some cases it may trigger defensive aggression. Aggression can also be seen in ill health due to irritability lowering the threshold at which the dog will do so (see Fig. 39). This may occur even in historically mild-mannered or tolerant dogs. Medical management of pain and alleviation of symptoms will help minimize this. The client can also be counselled in how to manage the behaviour whilst the dog recovers in the short term (see Box 12.1).

If the illness resolves but the dog persists with strongly fearful behaviour or aggression the client should be referred to an accredited behaviourist. If the dog is showing aggression due to illness or pain that cannot be alleviated and is terminal the issue of quality of life needs to be considered.

Desensitization and counter-conditioning to procedures

A programme of counter-conditioning may be indicated for procedures that may need to be performed long term, e.g. injections in diabetic dogs. How to perform this will need to be adapted to each procedure (see Chapter 7). The principles and how they can be applied to a specific example are outlined in Table 48. The intrinsically unpleasant nature of some medical interventions may make this challenging. However, it may help the dog learn the intervention is not as bad as they anticipate or may help if the pleasure of the anticipated food or other reward outweighs the distress caused. Even where the dog remains concerned by it the training can lessen this to some degree. Guidance from an accredited behaviourist may be needed if the nurse or technician is not confident of adapting this example to different procedures or the dog is showing higher level concern even at the start.

Confinement or cage rest

If a dog requires extended periods of rest, such as after orthopaedic procedures, the behavioural implications need to be considered both on welfare grounds and for their potential long-term impact. Where even relatively short periods of rest are needed during a puppy's sensitive periods it will be important to prevent this interfering with normal development. Examples of the types of problems that may arise due to extended cage rest are discussed in Table 49.

Clarifying instructions

When prescribing cage rest, confinement or restricted exercise it is important to make to clear to the client exactly what is required to avoid misinterpretation or over-zealous application. Box 12.2 identifies key points for clarification.

Stimulation

Boredom can be alleviated by providing the dog with environmental enrichment and entertainment.

Table 48. An example programme of desensitization and counter-conditioning to insulin injections.

Principle	Example application
Make current treatment distinctly different to treatment when training	If a dog has been diagnosed as diabetic the injections need to start being given straight away. Each real injection will cause distress and undermine any attempt to teach the dog to be less concerned by them. This effect can be lessened by making injections currently given very different from those given during training, e.g. given by a different person or in a different room. One option is for training to be performed by the owner whilst the dog is still being injected by practice staff during stabilization. Alternatively the client can use a signal of some sort to distinguish them, such as putting a bandanna on the dog when giving real injections but not when training. The distinction must be very obvious to the dog.
Teach the dog to accept the equipment used in the treatment	Get out the syringe and a dummy bottle of insulin. Leave them where the dog can see but not reach them. Ensure the dog can leave the room if he wants to. If he is showing fear or stress move them further away (see Box 11.3). Once he is no longer worried by them at all engage him in something pleasurable for a few minutes, e.g. play. Put the equipment away as soon as the play/training is over. Repeat four or five times a day until the dog looks excited when they are brought out.
Teach the dog to accept the preparatory steps used in the treatment	Get out the syringe and dummy insulin. Draw up some dummy insulin in the syringe. If the dog looks worried this process may need to be broken down into smaller steps. If he is happy the owner can play as above. Put the equipment away as soon as the play/training is over. Repeat four or five times a day until the dog no longer worries at all when the dummy insulin is drawn up.
Teach the dog to accept dummy treatment	Get out and draw up the dummy insulin. Gently hold the dog's scruff then, as long as he is not showing fear or stress, then play as above. Repeat as above. Once he looks excited at this hold his scruff and the syringe next to it without actually making the injection then play. In some cases each step may need to be smaller, e.g. initially gently hold the scruff without holding the syringe, then hold the syringe next to the scruff, then pair the two. The initial sensation of an injection can be simulated by gently touching with the tip of a cocktail stick.
Perform the procedure with the counter-conditioning	By this stage it should be possible to perform all preparatory steps without the dog being at all concerned. When needing to actually perform the procedure ask someone to help with counter-conditioning. For food-motivated dogs this may by smearing a little of the dog's food ration (within treatment protocols) on to a spoon and letting the dog lick it off as the injection is made. In play-motivated dogs it may be by showing the dog a toy and asking him to sit and wait for it as the injection is made, then giving it to him as soon as it is. This is the ultimate step. The previous steps simply maximize the chance this step will work by keeping the dog relaxed right up until the point of injection.

Table 49. Problems that can arise from extended cage rest.

Problem	Prevention
Breakdown or lack of toilet training	Dogs that are prevented from eliminating outdoors risk a breakdown in toilet training. If this occurs during very early puppy development the opportunity to train effectively may be missed, creating a long-term problem (see Chapter 14).
Boredom	Prolonged lack of stimulation or activity will result in boredom, which the dog will invariably develop behavioural strategies to alleviate. These may include vocalization or other attention-seeking strategies, attempts to escape or compulsions such as self-mutilation.
Breakdown in social behaviour	Being isolated from people or other dogs may cause existing social behaviour to break down. Prolonged cage rest during developmental periods may result in failure to properly socialize or habituate, causing irreversible damage.

Box 12.2. Points for clarification when advising a client on giving cage rest.

- Which part(s) of the body are to be rested?
- Can the dog be taken outside for elimination and does he need support to do so?
- Is the dog permitted to stand?
- Is the dog permitted to put weight on a rested limb? If so for how long?
- Is the dog permitted to walk? If so for how long?
- Is the dog permitted to run? If so for how long?
- Can the dog be permitted to jump?
- Can the dog be permitted to swim?
- How can this be increased over the duration of prescribed rest?

Methods will need to be selected and modified according to the condition being treated. However, even the most sedentary dog can be given some stimulation and the importance of this for emotional wellbeing, on-going behavioural management and recovery must not be under-estimated.

Tables 50 and 51 suggest examples of environmental enrichment and entertainment. This is of particular importance during developmental periods. Puppies still in their socialization and habituation period still need to be exposed to life's experiences if the efforts to treat their physical problem now is not to be in vain due to later problems with behaviour. The needs of puppies in later developmental periods must also be considered as a lack of on-going socialization can still be very detrimental.

It is advisable to set specific times each day for these activities and ask the dog to perform a simple task before starting them, such as 'sit' or 'watch'.

This will make the games predictable and lessen the likelihood the dog will try to get attention at other times by vocalizing or performing attention-seeking behaviours.

Elizabethan collars

When fitting an Elizabethan collar it is important to warn clients of the possible effect on behaviour. If the collar obscures the dog's ability to see someone approaching or their body language this may lead to increased defensive aggression. The collar may also prevent appeasement or withdrawal, or the dog's perception of it, increasing the likelihood he will opt for 'fight' rather than 'flight'.

Outside visits

The need to maintain visits outside for elimination must be impressed on the owner, other than

---

Table 50. Environmental enrichment during cage rest.

Stimulation	Description
Positioning crate: company	Move the crate or play pen to where the family is, assuming the dog shows signs of wanting to be with them. This can include sleeping upstairs if that is what they are used to and are small enough to be carried.
Positioning crate: outdoors	Put the crate outside for periods in good weather or position near a window in bad. This is contraindicated where the dog will try to jump at wildlife or is territorial. Ensure the dog does not overheat.
Car rides or buggies	Take the dog for car rides or take smaller dogs out in a buggy (see Fig. 78).
Visitors	Human visitors that sit and interact with the dog can be beneficial. Old placid dogs that will help develop or maintain canine social interaction without inciting play or frustration are also useful.
Carry outdoors	Puppies in their developmental periods can often still be carried outdoors in the same way as unvaccinated puppies (see Chapter 9).
Habituation tapes	Very young puppies benefit from habituation tapes for sounds they will not have the opportunity to experience, e.g. lorries, car horns, countryside noises.

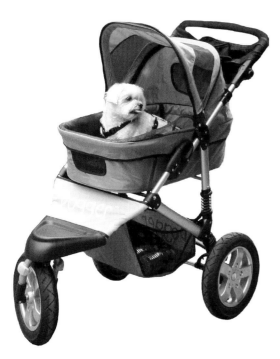

Fig. 78. Transporting a dog using a buggy (photograph courtesy of Dogquality.com).

where strictly contraindicated. This can be facilitated by placing the dog in a small crate for transportation to a confined outdoor area. Larger dogs can often be moved using specialized harnesses or hoists.

Cognitive Impairment

Cognitive functioning will deteriorate as the canine brain ages. This occurs through a number of processes as discussed in Chapter 2. Initial diagnosis of cognitive impairment as a cause for problem behaviour lies with the veterinary surgeon. However, owners may not immediately notice and so report the symptoms. It is therefore important for the veterinary nurse or technician to be aware of these so they can be brought to the vet's attention if seen or reported to them. The key symptoms are discussed in Chapter 2. Onset of brain ageing is often insidious with initially mild or intermittent behaviours. As time passes they become more frequent, consistent and intense. They often are not noticed by the owner until quite advanced. Brain ageing can occur in any dog over 8 years of age. It is more prevalent in dogs from 11 years onwards. Onset is not linked to breed, body size or life expectancy. It is typical for behaviours to start mildly and become more intense or frequent as the condition progresses.

Veterinary treatments

Brain ageing is caused by permanent changes to the structure of the brain and the way in which nerves transmit messages around the body. Treatment is therefore limited to slowing progression rather than a cure. Treatment is most effective when it is given at an early stage.

The veterinary surgeon may prescribe medication, nutraceuticals or dietary changes to slow progression.

Table 51. Entertainment for cage-rested dogs.

Method	Discussion
Training	Basic training can and should be maintained, especially in puppies and young dogs. The inability to attend classes does not mean the owner is unable to continue with most exercises at home. If they are already enrolled in classes they should be encouraged to still attend without the dog for guidance on the on-going training of their dog at home.
Massage	Gentle massage can provide interaction and promote relaxation. Observe the dog's body language to determine if he is finding it enjoyable. Stop briefly and see if he initiates you to start again.
Cuddling	Simply lying with the dog and cuddling can be relaxing and satisfying for the dog.
Hand wrestling	Depending on the dog, playing by patting the dogs paws and face can be enjoyable without it getting out of hand.
Scent games	If the dog is allowed to walk then hiding food in the crate can encourage seeking by scent. The dog can also be taught to identify items bearing a specific scent, which can then be applied to various items for the dog to find for a reward. Such games may be able to played on a lead outdoors once the dog is allowed to walk for specific periods of time.
Feeding	All food should be fed via an activity feeder of some kind. Exactly what is used will depend on the dog's preference and the type of rest needed. Kongs, treat balls, kibble dispensers, puzzle toys and muffin tins all ensure that the dog spends the maximum time eating their normal ration. Freezing wet food or soaked dry food in Kongs and other toys makes it last longer.
Toys	Rotate passive toys such as chews and chew toys, stuffed Kongs and puzzle games. When reintroducing a toy add to its interest by giving it a new smell. This can be by storing it somewhere smelly or adding an essential oil or other edible substance such as vanilla, aniseed, lavender or mint.
Simple tricks	Play the 'three cup' trick with the dog.

This can be supported with environmental management and enrichment.

Environmental management

The effects of memory loss and confusion can be reduced by keeping the things that are important to the dog in the same place. For example, feeding bowls and beds should not be moved and should be sited in easily and continually accessible areas. Avoid moving furniture. Maintaining routines for feeding, walking etc. also avoid confusion and anxiety. Elimination accidents can be minimized with regular visits outside, supervised to ensure the dog does so. Ensure stressors are kept to a minimum.

Enrichment

Cognitive decline can be slowed by actively stimulating the dog's brain throughout the day. Examples of how to do this are listed in Table 52.

Sensory Impairment

Blind dogs

Dogs that do not have functional use of their eyes, whether congenitally or due to illness or trauma, can still lead active fulfilled lives with some modifications to their environment and interactions with others. When a dog's sight fades gradually they usually adjust as the disability progresses. They are also usually left with some ability to determine light and shade and so often are not completely without sight. However, where the sight loss is sudden, such as due to acute illness and trauma, or where a dog has undergone a bilateral enucleation, some may initially find this very stressful and need much more guidance and support. Existing problem behaviour may also become more prominent or difficult to manage following loss of sight. The usual methods for reducing anxiety such as use of pheromones, 'escape to safety', consistent management and handling and pharmacological support can be employed to help the dog through the period of adjustment (see Chapter 7). Additional specialized methods are as follows.

Table 52. Examples of enrichment to slow cognitive decline.

Enrichment	Discussion
Toys	Provide toys the dog finds stimulating. Interaction can be encouraged through use of food inside or smeared on the toy, interaction with the dog when he plays or toys that make noises.
Training	Practise known tricks and commands to maintain neural function. Keep training short. Give strong clear commands or signals and high-value rewards. Consider the effect of any sensory impairment on the dog's ability to sense commands and rewards.
Scenting games	Hide highly smelly titbits for the dog to seek out. If the dog is fed dry food his daily ration can also be fed in this way. However, if doing so it is important to observe to make sure he remembers to eat it.
Interaction	Provide short frequent periods of play or communication throughout the day.
Exercise	Provide short regular walks, typically 10–15 min two to three times a day, depending on condition. This maintains blood flow to the brain and reduces night-time restlessness.

Table 53. Using remaining senses to assist navigation in blind dogs.

Sense	Use
Smell	Smells can be applied to obstacles or surfaces to help the dog locate and identify them. Application needs to be maintained or topped up so they become predictable to the dog. Everyday scents can be employed such as scented polish, perfumes, fabric freshener or very small quantities of nontoxic essential oils. If they cannot be applied directly to the surface they can be applied to a cloth that is attached to the obstacle. Scented discs designed for this purpose are also commercially available. Position scents at the dog's head height.
Touch	Mats or runners can be used to mark key locations or pathways such as doors, routes across a room and feeding stations. Artificial whiskers can help the dog 'feel' obstacles ahead or to the side before he bumps into them (see Fig. 79). Artificial or real plants can provide a soft signal he is approaching something, e.g. a tree, gate or table.
Sound	Leaving a radio or other clearly identifiable sound on permanently in the room the dog sleeps in helps with orientation when waking from sleep. Attaching small bells to major obstacles can help warn the dog before impact and help with identification. Bells attached to other members of the household (including humans) enables the dog to monitor their whereabouts. Wind chimes by external doors that are often left open will help with location.

Environmental management

A blind dog's ability to navigate around their home and garden will be greatly helped by keeping furniture in the same place and avoiding clutter on floors. They are then able to learn the position of obstacles they need to avoid. Table legs, cupboards etc. can be padded with bubble wrap or pipe insulation to prevent pain or injury, which may deter movement in the future, whilst the dog is learning to get around. It is wise to avoid picking up a blind dog where possible and if unavoidable to always put him down in the same place such as his bed so he knows where he is. The dog's ability to navigate can also be aided by employing their other senses. How to do so is discussed in Table 53.

A blind dog's ability to perceive and avoid hazards is compromised and so steps must be taken to protect him from harm. Barriers need to be erected around ponds, pools etc. Dog gates across doorways and at the top and bottom of staircases can prevent straying,

access to rooms that are not 'dog proofed' and accidents.

Blind dogs will often quickly cope with walking up stairs under supervision but many will be reluctant to walk down, especially small dogs. They cannot confidently see where the next step is and so will need to take a 'leap of faith'. Short runs of steps, such as a few steps into a garden, can be modified with a ramp to enable the dog to get up and down without aid. Plants, barriers or other objects can be used to prevent access to steps not covered by the ramp. The dog will usually learn more quickly if he is trained to walk up the ramp first to build confidence.

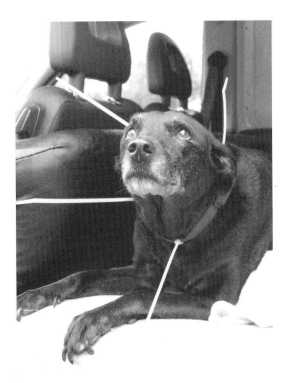

A barrier or other obstacles will prevent falling off the sides (see Fig. 80). Dogs that get on to beds or sofas can be provided with steps in the form of poufs or small tables so they can step or jump up and down two or three levels rather than having to make the transition in one.

Training

Blind dogs are still able to learn new commands, many of which can then be used to manage behaviour and build their confidence through communication. Useful commands to teach are outlined in Table 54. Blind dogs often respond well to use of a clicker for training. An accredited trainer can help with this.

Exercise

Blind dogs still need exercise. However, some may find walking in unfamiliar places worrying. Following the same route each day, using a hand target or target stick and the commands discussed above can help with this. Alternatively the dog can be transported to a familiar flat and obstacle-free exercise area by car, in the owner's arms or a dog buggy (see Fig. 78). Depending on the dog's recall he can be exercised off lead or on a long line. Great care should be taken when allowing interactions with other dogs

Fig. 79. Rufus: artificial whiskers to help a dog navigate (photograph courtesy of Laura Wyllie).

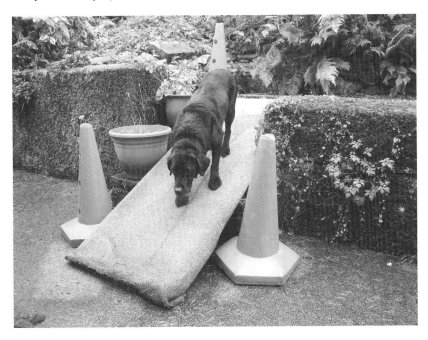

Fig. 80. Molly using a ramp designed to enable blind dogs to navigate short runs of steps (photograph courtesy of Graham Thompson).

Table 54. Useful commands to teach blind dogs.

Command	Use
Touch	To let the dog know he is about to be handled or touched.
Target	Teaching a dog to touch a hand, target stick or other implement enables them to be 'led' in unfamiliar settings.
Here	Teach the dog to navigate to a knocking sound. This can then be used to guide the dog to specific places.
Lift	To let the dog know he is going to be lifted up.
Left	To tell the dog to turn left to avoid walking into an obstacle.
Right	To tell the dog to turn right to avoid walking into an obstacle.
Stop	To tell the dog to stop to prevent him walking into an obstacle.
New recall signal	A verbal recall may be hard to locate in a busy place without the aid of sight. Teaching a recall to a new distinctive signal such as a whistle will help.

as the blind dog will not be able to read visual signals and so may not realize if another dog is being threatening. Only allow interaction with dogs known to be consistently friendly and use commands to intervene or control the interaction if needed.

Blind dogs can still enjoy games of tug or other contact games. You can play fetch with balls or other toys that are scented or make some kind of noise, e.g. have a bell inside or rattle. Ensure there are no obstacles and the game is always played in the same place. The dog can also be allowed to play with a weighted ball or a treat ball in a confined area such as a small room or a paddling pool with high rigid sides. They also enjoy games that involve finding or following scents, whether through informal games such as finding smelly food or kibble in a safe, flat and confined area, or more formal scent and tracking sports.

Deaf dogs

Dogs that are partially or profoundly deaf, whether congenitally or due to illness or trauma, generally cope very well providing their particular needs are accommodated.

Communication

The greatest hurdle to overcome with deaf dogs is communication. Humans are in the habit of and expect to communicate with dogs using words, as our preferred form of communication. However, this is our language and dogs are just as – if not more – able to learn what we want them to do from a visual or tactile signal as they are from a word. The type of signal used will depend on the individual dog and the circumstance. Options for visual signals are discussed in Table 55.

Waking a deaf dog

Touching a deaf dog unexpectedly, especially when sleeping, may startle him. Hearing dogs will no doubt have already sensed a person is there from footsteps, breathing or doors opening and closing. However, the deaf dog may be taken completely by surprise. Newly deaf dogs or dogs that are nervous or sensitive about being touched can be woken by placing a smelly food treat close to the nose and then crouching within the dog's line of sight ready for when they open their eyes.

Confident dogs can also be taught to expect good things when woken by touch to lessen the startle. The owner should start by gently touching various parts of the body whilst the dog is focused on them, to determine where he is comfortable being touched. Aim for those parts of the body that will be accessible most of the time e.g. top of the head, shoulder blades, mid-back or flank. The owner can then teach the dog being touched there is a predictor of good things. They should start when the dog is awake and focused on the owner. Hold out a treat and as the dog takes it gently touch the body part. If using a lateral location, practise touching on both sides. Repeat this five times, a few times each day for 3 days. If the dog is completely comfortable with this they can then progress to touching and treating when the dog is distracted and finally when asleep. Through repetition the dog will learn to expect a treat when touched in this way and so reduce the likelihood he will be startled.

Visitors should be asked not to touch the dog until he has been introduced to them and is familiar with their smell. They must then all follow the trained way of touching or using food to wake or seek his attention.

Table 55. Visual signals that can be used with deaf dogs.

Source	Discussion
Hand signals	Hand signals can follow an established sign language, such as American sign language, British sign language or traditional obedience or gundog signals (see Additional Resources). Alternatively they can be improvised by the owner. The signal needs to be distinctive from everyday hand and body movements. Dogs that are not very observant may need obvious and expansive gestures. Nervous dogs may respond better to more subtle signals.
Lights	Torches or outside lights can be used to recall dogs from the garden after dark. Torches can be used in the dark to get a deaf dog's attention or coded to become commands, e.g. two flashes means 'sit'. Lights can also be used as a reward marker in the same way as a clicker (see Chapter 7). High-powered laser pointers are visible in daylight but care needs to be taken with their use due to the risk of damage to the retina.
Touch	Touches to parts of the body can be used as commands. This is particularly useful for the initial 'look at me' command although care should be taken when using touch commands with a dog that is not focused on the handler. Teaching the dog not to startle when touched is discussed further in the text.
Vibration	Stamping on the floor or banging a door can create enough vibration to attract attention, enabling the use of other visual commands. However, the force needed to do so may worry nervous animals. Collars that vibrate can also be used for recall or 'look at me' commands. However, these need to be introduced carefully and the individual dog's response to them assessed as some may find them worrying. Great care must be taken when selecting these as electronic pulse collars are also often euphemistically described as 'vibration' collars. True vibration collars do not have prongs.

Safety

The deaf dog is at greater risk from some hazards, such as cars or lawn mowers, as he may not hear them approaching. Therefore this needs to be kept in mind when supervising him. Teaching the dog to routinely return to the owner for rewards on command and rewarding the dog when he spontaneously does so will reduce the chance he will wander off. It can also help to attach a bell to the dog's collar so the owner is aware of where he is and can find him if he does so.

Deaf dogs can be allowed to run off lead in places free of hazards providing their reliability for regularly looking at the owner for commands is as good as their recall.

Additional Resources

Barry Eaton (2005) *'Hear Hear'. A book on living with and training a deaf dog.* Pine Cottage, Chilbolton, UK.

'Basic Sign Language' fact sheet by Morag Heirs MSc MA(SocSci)(Hons.) PGCAP. Available at: http://www.apbc.org.uk/system/files/private/advice_sheet_5_-_teaching_basic_sign_language.pdf

Blind Dog Info: A web-based resource for owners of blind or partially sighted dogs. Available at: http://www.blinddog.info

Deaf Dog Network: A UK-based information and support group for owners of deaf dogs. Includes images of useful signs. Available at: http://www.deafdognetwork.org.uk

Deaf Dog Education Action Fund (DDEAF): USA-based resource for owners of deaf dogs. Available at: http://www.deafdogs.org

Helen Zulch, Peter Baumber and Sian Ryan (2014): No walks? No worries! Maintaining well-being for dogs on restricted exercise. Hubble & Hattie, Veloce Publishing Ltd, Dorchester

13 Managing Behaviour During Life Changes

Dogs are creatures of habit. Most changes in a dog's life are imposed either by circumstance or their human carers. Well-balanced easy-going dogs will generally adjust to these changes without too much concern, especially where it does not involve a change in their primary social companions. However, being aware of the potential impact of these changes can help owners take steps to minimize this, especially in dogs that show signs of worry around new things or that are prone to fear or stress.

Adoption by a New Owner

The dog's primary attachment is to its social companions. As such the life change that has the greatest impact on a dog is being transferred to new owners.

Reasons for rehoming are complex. They may be heartfelt and genuinely unavoidable. They may be frivolous and indifferent. They may be as a result of the dog being rescued from neglectful or abusive owners. Humans would view each of these differently. However, they are all the same to the dog. He has lost the person he had formed a social bond with, whether they were loving and kind or distant and neglectful.

Multiple changes of social companion

A dog's carer may change multiple times. Some of these may be true 'ownership' as humans would term it, i.e. people who are not only caring for the dog at the moment but who intend to keep the dog for the rest of his life. They may also be transient such as a period in kennels or a foster home. If the dog spends more than a couple of weeks with any social group he will normally form a bond with them and so will be affected by any subsequent change. Even staff changes in rescue centres can be seen as a loss to the dog where particular attachments have been made. Each change in the person caring for the dog therefore has to be considered a rehoming when looking at the dog's history.

Settling in

How long it takes a dog to settle into a new home is very variable. Anecdote and informal research suggests it takes most dogs 2–3 weeks to accept a new home as permanent, after which there are often changes in behaviour, which may be for better or for worse. However, this is not always the case and dogs that have been rehomed multiple times, that are highly anxious or are traumatized may take longer.

Some dogs may still form an attachment to their new people during this initial adjustment period, whereas others may remain cautious until settled or beyond. Once a bond is formed some dogs may then become overly attached to the new owner, in fear they too may then suddenly disappear. How long it takes for a dog to learn a new owner is now their permanent social companion is difficult to measure. It is known for dogs that start by following the owner everywhere and show distress as soon as they leave the house to gradually settle over time. However, this is very variable depending on the circumstances, the dog's character, past experiences, number of rehomings and whether the problem behaviour is inadvertently encouraged or aggravated in some way.

Choosing the rescue dog

Although prospective owners are often very keen to meet the dog being rehomed it is critical that they are given background information regarding the dog's character and history before doing so. Once a new owner sees a dog and their heart goes out to them they may stop objectively considering whether they are the right person for the dog. Repeated rehoming tends to adversely affect the dog's behaviour and so ensuring the new owner is the right one is critical.

Prospective owners need to be made aware of the dog's needs and any issues that he has. Many people relinquish dogs due to problem behaviour. The new owner must be aware of these problems and what will be entailed in overcoming them on a practical and real level. It is common for prospective owners to have the very best of intentions or to quickly become emotionally attached to the dog, but to be in no better a position to support the dog than the previous one was. The dog is then invariably rehomed again once reality hits home.

The transition

Once the decision has been made that a new owner will adopt a dog, both parties to the human bargain are often keen to make the transition as soon as possible. However, it is hugely beneficial if the dog can be given the opportunity to meet their new owner a few times before adoption.

If the dog is still in the previous home this can be accommodated by the new owner calling around each day for a few days and feeding, playing with or taking the dog for a walk. This allows the dog to build trust with the new stranger before being removed from the old, making the transition far less traumatic. If a dog is in a rescue centre there will usually be a delay between the dog being chosen and being collected, due to the need for completion of paperwork and home checks. This offers the opportunity for new owners to meet and play with or walk their new dog a few times before taking him home. Some rescues do not require home checks and may suggest the dog is taken home as soon as he has been chosen to reduce the stress induced by the kennel environment or to make space for another dog. If the dog is not eating or is showing acute stereotypies this may be justified. However, for a dog that is relatively settled a sudden transition may be more stressful than a few more days in kennels.

Environment

Dogs primarily rely on scent for identifying people and safe environments. Transferring scents between old and new can therefore be beneficial. New owners can impregnate cloths with their scent by wearing or sleeping with them and then leave them with the dog whilst awaiting rehoming. These cloths and a small piece of the dog's used bedding should then accompany the dog to his new home.

Adaptil™ spray in the car and diffusers in the new home can help promote positive associations on arrival. An Adaptil™ collar can ensure the benefit of the pheromone is with the dog wherever he goes (see Chapter 7).

A den will give the dog a refuge in the new home if he feels the need to withdraw. This can both reduce fear and anxiety by providing an 'escape to safety' and minimize the risk of aggression by providing a clear 'flight' option. How to set up a den is discussed in Chapter 7. Introduce the dog to his den by feeding him in there and placing toys and snacks in it. Initially position the den where the dog can get away from people without being isolated. If he chooses to stay with people rather than sit in the den it can be moved closer to the family area so the dog can have the best of both worlds. The dog must always be left in peace in the den other than in emergencies.

When first bringing the dog home the owner should take him to the place in which he will need to urinate and allow him to explore. It may help if this area has already been 'seeded' by another dog urinating there by bringing a friend's dog around – or a sample of his urine.

Interactions

The dog should be allowed to set the pace for the interactions and should not be overwhelmed in his first few days. It is tempting for new owners to want to show off their new dog but this will set the settling in period back in shy dogs.

Rehoming often fails due to the dog showing higher levels of threat such as growling and snapping in the early days. This is most likely to be due to fear and elevated stress levels causing the dog to behave defensively. Owners therefore need to be made aware of low-level canine stress and threat signals so they can identify these and withdraw before they escalate to higher threat (see Fig. 21).

The dog should be the only one to initiate interactions for the first few days. As they then become more relaxed the owner can start to do so, providing the dog has been comfortably interacting so far. The owner can test whether the dog is enjoying this attention by petting then briefly stopping whilst keeping the hand close to see if the dog encourages them to continue by nuzzling or pawing. They should always respect the dog's attempt to withdraw, or request for them to withdraw using appeasing or threat signals.

Routines

Dogs are creatures of habit and so routines help them feel secure. Following daily routines for the things that are important to the dog such as feeding, walking and play time will help the dog settle into his new home more quickly. They should ideally be maintained 7 days a week for the initial settling in period. They can be modified at weekends once the dog is more established.

Leaving the dog alone

It is best for the dog not to be left alone at all for the first few days to give him the opportunity to adjust to the new environment. He can then be familiarized to being left gradually over the next couple of weeks as summarized in Box 13.1.

Where the dog sleeps at night is a personal decision. It is fine for the dog to sleep in the owner's bedroom or even on their bed if this is what they would like. The only exception to this is if the dog shows aggression around the bed, in which case the client needs to be referred to an accredited behaviourist. The dog should always have access to his den if he would prefer to withdraw. If the owner would prefer the dog to sleep elsewhere in the house it is advisable to start by initially settling him somewhere he is not totally isolated and then gradually moving him away as he settles in and become more confident. This is especially true if the dog is showing signs of being highly attached due to fear of further abandonment. In this case the client can start with the dog's bed in the owner's bedroom or just outside of the room with the door open, and a baby gate across if needed. He can then gradually be moved further away.

Introduction to existing pets

If the client already has other pets, the likelihood the new dog will get on with the existing pets and vice versa needs to be carefully considered. If there are any concerns but the owners are still keen to adopt they should be referred to an accredited behaviourist to further discuss prognosis for success.

How to introduce a new dog to an existing dog, assuming neither has concerns around other dogs, is discussed below. The principles for introducing a cat-friendly dog to a dog-friendly cat are the same as introducing a new puppy to a cat (see Box 10.8).

Changes to the Household

New baby

Preparation

Steps can start to be taken to prepare a dog for the arrival of a new baby as soon as the pregnancy is confirmed. Ways to do this are summarized in Box 13.2. These will help reduce the number of new things the dog needs to adjust to when the baby arrives.

If the dog has any training or behavioural concerns it is best to address these as soon as possible. The arrival of the baby may aggravate some problems, such as fearful, anxious or attention-seeking behaviour. It may also change the importance of them. People are far less willing to tolerate a dog that snaps if there are children in the house.

Box 13.1. Teaching a new dog to settle when left.

- The dog ideally should not be left alone at all for the first few days.
- Advise the client to take the dog for a walk or play for a while before leaving for the first time. They should also make sure he is not hungry and does not need to eliminate.
- The dog should be given a safe chew or food toy.
- Advise the owner to establish a leaving routine that the dog can learn predicts being left, in a way in which he is comfortable, e.g. turning on a radio or saying 'time to go.'
- The dog should initially be left for about 15 min. If possible the dog should be video recorded or monitored via a webcam.

- The owners should greet calmly on their return. They should never punish or talk sternly to the dog when they return, whatever he has done, and should not ignore him as this is punishing to the dog. It can therefore cause rather than prevent separation problems.
- If he is settling without problem they can gradually increase how long he is left over the coming days and weeks.
- If the dog is showing signs of distress at being left the owner can try initially leaving for shorter periods, e.g. 2–3 min. If he is still distressed, refer the client to an accredited behaviourist.

Poor recall or lead pulling can also be much more of a problem when there are children with the owner on walks.

Introductions

As soon as the baby is born ask a family member to take something with the baby's own scent on home to the dog. Allow him to sniff but not grab, play with or lay on this.

When the mother initially comes home after the birth of the baby she should ask someone else to carry the baby into the house so she can greet the dog unhindered. The dog can then be allowed to sniff the baby and his accoutrements. Use commands and rewards if the dog wants to greet or interact in an inappropriate way. It is essential the dog is not punished or excluded during early introductions to avoid creating anxiety around the baby. If the owners are at all concerned they can have the dog on a lead and jolly him away at the first sign he is concerned.

On-going management

The first few weeks with a new baby, especially a first baby, can be a little chaotic. However, the client should try as best they can to keep to their dog's routines. If walks will be difficult at first then it may be possible to enlist help from friends or employ a dog walker to ensure they are not missed. Meals should be maintained at the normal times and time set aside for interaction so the dog does not feel pushed out. Baby gates and/or time-consuming treats such as chews and Kongs can help settle the dog without the need to exclude him behind a solid barrier at feeding and changing times.

Although a few dogs may be jealous or anxious around a new baby at first, it is rare that this causes aggression. There is a very slight risk the baby may trigger a predatory response in some dogs, due to baby noises and movements being similar to those of wounded prey. This is exceptionally rare, and invariably makes headline news when it happens. However, the tragedy that arises means all parents should be aware the risk exists and seek help if they are at all concerned by their dog's behaviour towards the baby. Key factors to look for are summarized in Box 13.3. If an owner observes any of these behaviours the dog should be kept apart from the baby until an accredited behaviourist can assess him properly.

The golden rule with babies in all circumstances is that the dog is never left alone with the baby. This is discussed further below.

Growing up

Most dogs love children and have a natural instinct to be gentle with and protective of them. However, a small proportion of dogs may start to become concerned once the baby starts to become mobile. The risk of a bite is at its highest in the period between when the baby starts crawling until he is old enough to reliably do as he is asked when handling and being around the dog. This applies to all dogs as even the gentlest family dog can be pushed to behave defensively if a child unwittingly hurts him.

Toddlers must never be allowed to mishandle the dog, however tolerant he may seem to be. Owners need to be made aware of canine communication signals that indicate he is unhappy and how this can escalate to aggression if the dog feels lower level signals are not effective at making the child stop.

The dog must be provided with an 'escape to safety' (see Chapter 7) that is accessible at all times so he can withdraw if he is finding a child's behaviour too much. The child must be taught from as soon as they can crawl not to approach the dog in this place, just as they are taught not to touch an electrical socket or hot stove. Depending on the size of the dog and layout of the house it may be possible to site the escape somewhere the child cannot get to, such as behind a barrier the dog can jump over, facing close to a wall so the dog can get in but not the toddler or raised up above the toddler's head height.

The child must also be prevented from approaching the dog when he is eating or chewing a bone. As soon as the child can stand and follow directions he can be involved in feeding, playing with and training the dog under direct and continuous supervision. For example, the child can throw the ball for a dog that is sitting politely to wait for it, and can toss the treat on the floor when the dog has obeyed a command. Once the child can walk he or she can place the dog's bowl of food on the floor after the dog has been asked to sit by the owner, and then walk away before the dog is released. This teaches both the dog and the child the rules for interaction. The child will learn to use commands and rewards rather than manipulation to control a dog. The dog will learn to respect and be motivated to obey the child's commands.

New person

Ideally a dog will have the opportunity to get to know and form a bond with a new person before they move into their home, although this is not always the case. Relaxed and confident dogs may take it in their stride. However, worried dogs may be unsettled by it.

The existing owner must ensure they still spend time with their dog and maintain their bond. However, the dog's bond with the new person can be helped by them taking over important care roles such as feeding and walking the dog. They can also set time aside each day to play with and train the dog using rewards such as play and treats.

The dog must be provided with an 'escape to safety' (see Chapter 7) so he can withdraw from the new person if he is worried. The person should be taught to read the dog's signals and to respect these. He or she should also regularly test if the dog is enjoying fuss in the early days by stopping briefly to see if the dog nudges or paws to encourage them to resume.

Loss of a household member

Loss of a household member, whether dog or human, can be very unsettling for a dog. The common symptoms of canine grief are summarized in Box 13.4. These will probably be the same whatever the cause of the loss, i.e. bereavement, separation or rehoming of another dog.

Bereavement

It can sometimes help to allow the dog to see the deceased before they are taken for cremation or burial. This helps them understand where they have gone and may reduce behaviour associated with trying to find them or waiting for them to come back. However, it is also possible this may distress the dog especially where it is the body of another dog that has been euthanized. It is therefore advisable to disguise the euthanasia of the other dog at home by taking the remaining dog for a walk for the duration of the vet's visit and not allowing the remaining dog to see the euthanized dog's body at the practice.

Support during grieving

Dogs, like people, do normally recover after a period of grieving. Ways in which they can be helped through the grieving process are summarized in Table 56.

Where the loss of a canine family member leaves two or more dogs behind there may be a change in the relationship between the remaining dogs. Alliances may change and established agreements over who controls or wins resources may need to be re-established. In most cases this is resolved by the dogs with posturing and appeasing. However, where it becomes protracted, one dog becomes excessively controlling or it leads to higher level aggression (e.g. growling, snarling or fights), then the help of an accredited behaviourist will be required. This should be sought as soon as possible to avoid the behaviour becoming a habit.

New dog

Dogs are social creatures and so the introduction of a new puppy or older dog will often be trouble free. However, it is always wise to manage the introductions carefully to avoid triggering any conflict, especially over valued resources, which may be hard to undo later.

Whether to get a new dog

The first consideration is whether a new dog should be introduced at all. It is surprising how commonly owners will acquire a new dog when their existing dog is fearful or aggressive to unfamiliar dogs. Some suggest they feel it may help the dog overcome their problems. Others assume the dogs will be fine once they get to know each other. Both of these may be true in some cases. However, this will entirely depend on why the existing dog is showing problem behaviour to others. Clients with dogs that are problematic around other dogs should therefore be advised to have the existing dog assessed by an accredited behaviourist to evaluate what the likely outcome will be before

---

Box 13.4. Common symptoms of grief at the loss of a companion.

- Loss of appetite.
- Increase in sleep.
- Lack of enthusiasm for normal activities, e.g. play, walks.
- Restlessness or aimless wandering, often looking for the departed member.
- Increased vocalization or attention seeking.

Table 56. Ways to support a dog during the grieving process.

Method	Discussion
Adaptil™	Pheromones can help reduce anxiety and so ease the transition
Activities	Dogs that become solitary will need more human play and interaction. Periods of play, walks or attention that used to be given by the absent member need to be performed by someone else.
Play dates	If a dog has lost his only canine companion and is sociable, arranging walks or play dates with other dogs will maintain canine companionship and interaction.
Familiarizing to being left alone	The loss of a canine companion may mean the dog has to be left alone when he is not used to it. He therefore needs to be familiarized to this gradually over a period of a few weeks to prevent it from causing problems.
Routines	Routines should be maintained to minimize the impact of the changes.
Scent	Keeping items with the lost family member's scent on until the dog seems to lose interest in them will help the transition. This can include unwashed bedding from another dog or worn clothing from a person.
Eating	Entice an anorexic dog to eat using favourite foods or by warming it. However, avoid hand feeding or making too much fuss in case this becomes a habit.
Medication	In extreme cases medication may help. This should be discussed with the vet.

---

acquiring the new dog. They can also advise on and supervise the introduction process.

Initial introductions – adult dogs

Assuming both dogs are friendly, adult dogs are best initially introduced on neutral territory. The client should avoid going anywhere the existing dog has had an unpleasant experience with another dog. If the new dog has been adopted from a rescue they may be able to offer an exercise paddock for this purpose. Allow the dogs to greet and play as they would with any other unfamiliar dog.

If the dogs need to be transported from the meeting place to the home by car it is best that they are separated to avoid forcing the dogs too close to each other at this early stage. Either use two cars or, if this is impossible, separate them in covered crates.

Once home the dogs should be allowed to meet in the garden. The existing dog should be taken into the garden first followed by the new dog. Trailing house lines are best used for the initial introduction. Toys or food should be removed. The owner should try not to intervene unless either dog starts to show higher level threat behaviour. If this occurs they should use jolly recalls or distractions rather than using the house lines to draw the dogs apart unless unavoidable. The client will then need to be referred to an accredited behaviourist for further advice on introductions. If introductions in the garden are successful this can then be transferred to the room in which the dogs will spend most of their time in the house.

Once the initial greetings are complete the new dog should be allowed to explore all parts of the house he will be allowed to access. If the existing dog seems bothered by this, one person should take him elsewhere and play with him or take him for a walk, whilst the new dog has the chance to get to know his new home.

The dogs should be provided with separate beds and feeding stations at first. It the client is not 100% confident of the dogs' interaction it is advisable that these are initially positioned either side of a secure baby gate the dogs cannot jump over. The dogs can then be in the same space but separated when eating or left alone. If they sleep in the client's bedroom their beds should initially be positioned on either side of the owner's bed. It also helps to spend time upstairs with the dogs whilst encouraging them to use their respective beds with a chew or stuffed Kong before the first night's sleep. Ideally the new dog's bed will be lined with an unwashed blanket from their previous home.

As a new dog settles in there may sometimes be jealousy or competition over resources such as toys, food, access to favourite resting places or owner interaction and attention. In the vast majority of cases dogs will work this out through low-level posturing and appeasing behaviour as they learn what the other is prepared to fight for. The owner can control conflict over interaction and attention by asking both dogs to always 'sit' for this to show it is their decision, not the dogs, when this is given. If one dog is being excessively controlling of all resources or the dogs are not able to resolve the disputes easily then the client will need to be referred to an accredited behaviourist. Help should be sought sooner rather than later to prevent conflict becoming a learnt expectation. The client should also be made aware that the dog's initial relationship may change as the new dog settles in and so to continue to observe behaviour over the coming weeks.

New cat

The dog's temperament around cats must be assessed before the decision is made to introduce a cat into a household. The cat's temperament around dogs must also be assessed. It is unfair to and potentially dangerous for both the cat and the dog if either of them are fearful of the other or the dog is predatory towards cats.

Cats are strongly territorial and even some dog friendly cats may regard a new dog as a potential predator. They must therefore be allowed to settle into the new home before being introduced to the dog. How to do this is outlined in Box 13.5.

House Move

A house move can be unsettling for a dog. This can be minimized as outlined in Box 13.6.

Kennels

Many dogs find periods in kennels concerning. This can be lessened as outlined in Box 13.7.

Box 13.5. Settling in a new cat.

- The cat should be allocated a room in the house and secured in there with his food and littler tray (at opposite ends of the room) for the first few days. The client should provide suitable hiding places, such as under furniture or on a high surface. A cardboard box placed on its side can provide an 'escape to safety' (see Chapter 7). The client should spend plenty of time with the cat over these few days.
- Both the dog and cat's scent can be transferred on to cloths, which can then be exchanged so they become familiar with each other's smell.
- The dog should be allowed to spend brief supervised periods on the other side of the cat's room so they can sniff each other under the door.
- After the first few days the cat should be allowed to explore the rest of the house whilst the dog is out on a walk. The client should encourage the

cat on to high surfaces using treats to ensure he knows where they are.
- When they are ready to be introduced the client should place a baby gate that the dog cannot jump over across the entrance to the cat's room. They must ensure the high surfaces the cat has been introduced to, both in the cat's safe room and elsewhere, are kept clear. These opportunities for the cat to withdraw should be maintained lifelong.
- The dog should be on a long trailing lead. Commands and rewards can be used to control any signs the dog looks likely to chase or greet inappropriately.
- The dog and cat should not be left alone together until the client knows they will not harm each other.
- If either party seems distressed or the dog shows any signs of predatory or chase behaviour the client should be referred to an accredited behaviourist.

Box 13.6. Reducing the impact of a house move.

- Friends or family can be asked to look after the dog(s) during the actual move to avoid the stress of this being associated with the new house.
- The dog's bed and feed station should be set up before the dog comes home.
- Advise clients not to wash bedding for a few days before and after the move.
- An Adaptil™ collar can be used starting a few days before the move and an Adaptil™ diffuser installed by the dog's bed in the new house.

- The dog's routines should be maintained as far as possible.
- If possible the dog should continue to be walked in the same places as he was before the move for a couple of weeks.
- Advise clients to find out if the new neighbours have dogs. If they do and all the dogs are friendly, it is advisable to initially introduce them away from the property to avoid fence running or frustration.

Box 13.7. Helping a dog to accept a period in kennels.

- Clients should choose kennels carefully. Choosing somewhere where the dog can stay on the same food, is taken out of the kennel regularly for exercise and elimination, and where interactions with other dogs are controlled and supervised will help reduce the impact of a period in kennels.
- It can help to leave the dog at the kennels for a few short visits before being left for an overnight stay for the first time.
- If the dog is not comfortable with other dogs he is best sited at the far end of a run of kennels to avoid other dogs passing by. Any mesh panels should be covered.

- An Adaptil™ collar or mild anxiolytics such as alpha-casozepine can help some dogs.
- Taking the dog's own unwashed bedding to the kennels may help him settle.
- Providing the kennel with toys and chews the dog enjoys and activity feeders can help reduce boredom.
- Staff should be made aware of any special needs the dog has, especially around human handling.
- On return the dog should be taken for a walk or into the garden to eliminate before going into the house to re-establish house training. Repeat if necessary.

PART 4
Addressing Problem Behaviour

When a puppy or dog develops problem behaviour the veterinary practice is often the first place the owner goes to for advice. Each practice therefore needs to develop a protocol for how such enquiries should be handled across the practice team.

The first consideration will always be elimination of physical cause. Once this has been addressed the next step will be deciding whether to address the problem in-house or to refer to a specialist. This section looks at how to determine the right approach for each type of problem behaviour, outlines advice that can be given in-house where appropriate and discusses the process of choosing and making a referral to a specialist when this is required.

14 Advising on Problem Behaviour

Medical Causes

When presented with a problem behaviour the first step should always be consideration and elimination of medical cause. In many cases this will be very straightforward. For example, a puppy that has always pulled on the lead and has no other problems is very unlikely to have a medical concern underpinning the behaviour. However, other problems that seem straightforward can sometimes have an unusual or insidious disease process behind them. Box 14.1 offers some real examples of this as food for thought.

Each practice will need to develop a protocol for deciding when a behaviour enquiry needs to have a veterinary examination prior to in-house advice or referral being made. Box 14.2 summarizes the key factors to take into account when developing this. Even where a veterinary examination has been conducted or the need has been eliminated the possibility of a medical cause needs to be kept in mind in case anything changes or any clinical signs come to light that were not initially apparent. The clinical signs and physical conditions that can underlie problem behaviour are summarized in Tables 6–8 (Chapter 2).

Deciding Whether to Refer

Once medical cause has been eliminated the next step is deciding whether to advise the client or refer them to an accredited behaviourist or trainer. Box 14.3 summarizes the types of cases that should always be referred to a specialist due to their complexity, the degree of practical support that will be needed and/or the risks associated with them. How to decide to whom to refer is discussed in Chapter 15. Whether to refer or advise in-house on other types of problem behaviour is discussed under each separate heading below.

The most likely source of information for making this decision will be the owner's description of their dog's problem behaviour. However, it is important to keep the client's limitations in giving accurate information in mind when doing so. Most will have limited behavioural knowledge and so may not be aware of problem behaviour, signs their dog is unhappy or even when he is being threatening. They may also sometimes find it hard to be objective, or may be embarrassed or worried about the consequences if they reveal certain information. It is also very easy for misunderstandings to occur. Ask specific questions and double-check you have understood correctly. Clarify any loose or colloquial terms. If you feel a client is being evasive, vague or inconsistent in their descriptions refer them to an accredited behaviourist. Whenever in doubt, always approach the accredited behaviourist you refer to for guidance.

House Soiling

Elimination

Voluntary control of elimination is achieved by 8 weeks. Once in place elimination is triggered by olfactory cues or extreme bladder pressure and is inhibited during sleep. The puppy will develop a preference to eliminate away from sleeping and eating areas. His preferred eliminatory medium and location is established by 16 weeks and is then hard to change. How to use this to maximize toilet training is discussed in Chapter 10.

Problems with elimination in the house may arise due to many reasons (see Box 14.4). The flow chart in Appendix 7 allows identification of cases that arise due to illness, fear or anxiety, separation issues or scenting. These should be referred to an accredited behaviourist.

Submissive urination in puppies and pubescent dogs is common and normally grown out of by about a year of age. Management involves taking the puppy outside or asking him to sit for greeting, not leaning over the puppy and ensuring owner behaviour is not inadvertently threatening.

Where the problem arises due to a lack of, or breakdown in, house training then the dog will need to undergo a new programme of house training. Practice staff can advise on this, if they feel confident to do so. The methods for teaching an adult dog to eliminate outdoors are principally the same as for a puppy, with greater emphasis on rewarding outdoor elimination. These are discussed in Chapter 10.

Initial Puppy Training Failure

Jumping up and mouthing

Puppy behaviours such as jumping up and mouthing may persist if the dog has not been effectively taught not to do so. Even if the owner is pushing the dog away or shouting at him, this may seem like a fun wrestling game to some dogs, encouraging them to do it. Some dogs also learn these behaviours often get attention when others fail and so use them to entice the owner to engage with them.

The flow chart in Appendix 8 identifies those cases that should be referred to an accredited behaviourist. If the behaviour only occurs in greeting, the methods discussed in Appendix 9 are usually sufficient to change the behaviour. However, if the client has tried these before and failed he or she should be referred to an accredited behaviourist.

Stealing

Dogs steal for many reasons. The flow chart in Appendix 10 identifies cases that should be referred to an accredited behaviourist. The remainder will most likely occur simply because the dog wants the item. The client therefore needs to be educated how to ensure their dog's needs for stimulation and exercise are fulfilled and that it is their responsibility to move food out of the dog's way when unsupervised (see Chapters 2 and 10).

Pulling on the Lead

Walking close to an owner on a lead is not a natural behaviour for a dog. Although dogs would normally stay within sight or earshot of their social companions they do not necessarily stay continually at their side. Dogs that pull on the lead therefore do so for the sole reason that they have not been taught or motivated not to.

Head collars and some designs of harness are often effective at helping to manage pulling. However, if the client would like their dog to walk on a loose lead without using these they need to be referred to an accredited trainer. Clients should be warned against using aversive methods such as check/choke chains, prong/pinch collars or slip leads. The reasons for this are expanded on in Chapter 7.

Failing to Come When Called

Dogs may fail to come when called for a number of reasons as outlined in Box 14.5. Making clients aware of these can often go a long way towards rectifying the problem. If the client needs more help they should be referred to an accredited trainer. Clients should be warned against using aversive methods such as static pulse electric shock, remote, 'stim' or E collars. The reasons for this are expanded on in Chapter 7.

Destructiveness and Chewing

Destructive behaviour can have many triggers. The flow chart in Appendix 11 identifies when the client should be referred to an accredited behaviourist. Those that remain will typically be due to boredom/lack of suitable exercise and stimulation, or attention seeking. The client therefore needs to be educated how to ensure their dog's needs for stimulation and exercise are fulfilled (see Chapters 2 and 10).

Digging

Digging is a natural behaviour rooted in ancestral creation of sleeping areas or storing of food items. Dogs will also dig for stimulation or exploration. Dogs that like to dig should be given a part of the garden in which it is safe and acceptable for them to dig. Suitable 'clean' substrates such as play pit sand, a mix of peat and wood shavings or bark chips can reduce mud being brought indoors. The dog can be encouraged to use that area by burying toys and chews in it and preventing access to other areas whilst the habit is developed. Once the dog has established his preferred digging area exclusion from other areas can usually be stopped.

Car Sickness

Canine car sickness can be miserable for both dog and owner. It is more common in puppies until the balance mechanisms in their ears have matured. However, it can persist in older dogs due to lack of habituation to car travel, associations between being in the car and nausea or anxiety about where the dog suspects he is going, e.g. to the vets. Symptoms of car sickness include restlessness, shaking, lip licking, yawning and hypersalivation as well as actual retching or vomiting. Methods for managing car sickness are outlined in Box 14.6.

Coprophagy

Coprophagy is common, although far from universal, in the domestic dog. Dogs may consume their own, other dogs or other species faeces, e.g. cat, sheep or horse. The possible causes for it are discussed in Box 14.7. The flow chart in Appendix 12 identifies when the client should be referred to the vet or an accredited behaviourist as appropriate. If a dog specifically seeks out another dog's faeces the health of that dog should also be considered. The remainder will most likely be due to boredom, habit or competition.

Habit can be broken by keeping the dog on lead until faeces is passed both in the garden and on walks. It can then be promptly removed. Using a cloth muzzle during elimination in the garden can also be useful for breaking the habit. The cloth muzzle should not be left on for longer than a few minutes and should not be used on walks as the dog cannot regulate his body temperature with it on. Cage muzzles often do not prevent the behaviour as the dog will eat through the muzzle.

Competition can be reduced by separating the coprophagic dog from others during elimination and not attempting to remove the faeces until the dog is distracted. Alternatively the dog can be taught a 'leave' command (see Appendix 6) and rewarded with very high-value treats for obeying. The client should start by standing very close to the dog when giving the command so his focus can be quickly be drawn on to the alternative reward. As the dog becomes reliable at obeying this command the owner can then gradually move away one step at a time, practising the command at each new distance until it is reliable then moving on to the next. This will take multiple sessions. The owner will need to supervise all potential defection opportunities throughout the training to make this a habit. If this is ineffective the client should be referred to an accredited behaviourist.

Treating Simple Fears and Phobias

Fears and phobias can arise due to a number of influences, as discussed in Chapters 2 and 6. The majority of these will need to be referred to an accredited

Box 14.7. Factors that may trigger or aggravate coprophagy.

- Prolonged confinement with faeces.
- Residual nutritional value in stools due to poorly digested diet.
- Illness or dietary inadequacies including hunger.
- Habit formed from observation of the dam or other dog's behaviour, or competition during development.
- Current boredom or habit formed from boredom during development.

- Interference by the owner, triggering competition or attention seeking.
- Competition over food with other dogs.
- Developmental oral frustrations (e.g. abnormal suckling or weaning) may lead to oral compulsions that are expressed in this way.
- Genetic tendency in some dogs due to evolution as a scavenger and to thrive on waste from human settlements.

behaviourist. However, fearful behaviour that only occurs in the veterinary practice or very specific fear or phobia of sounds such as fireworks may be able to be addressed under supervision of the practice in some cases.

Visiting the vets

Fear of going to the vets is very common and often arises due to unavoidable associations formed with feeling unwell or painful examinations or treatments. It is quite common for the veterinary practice to be the only place a dog shows fear or defensive aggression, although it is also possible for fear initially learned at the vets to then spread to other situations.

The first step is to confirm that the dog's fearful behaviour only occurs in the practice. If the client reports fear, aggression in any other situation or any other problem behaviour they should be advised to seek help from an accredited behaviourist.

How does treatment work?

It is impossible to prevent all unpleasant experiences at the vets. However, the dog's expectation of them can be reduced through a programme of desensitization and counter-conditioning.

Desensitization is the process whereby the dog learns to no longer be afraid of visiting the practice by arranging for him to do so in a completely non-threatening way. Counter-conditioning is the process of linking being at the practice to a pleasant emotion such as the pleasure triggered by food, play or fuss. Desensitization is needed before counter-conditioning as any fear the dog feels would prevent the pleasure generated by the food, etc., having the

desired effect. Counter-conditioning is needed after desensitization because desensitization can break down very easily after one unpleasant experience at the practice. This is less likely if the dog has had a lot of positively pleasant visits to the practice. These principles are discussed more in Chapter 7.

Identifying when the dog starts to be fearful

When performing this kind of training it is essential that dog's fear and stress levels are kept low so they cannot interfere with learning. The point at which each dog starts to worry therefore needs to be identified before the training can start. The likely points at which this may occur are listed in Box 14.8.

The client should start by identifying their own dog's signs of stress (see Box 11.3). They should then make a dummy run to the practice to see at what point on the journey the first signs of worry are seen.

Vets visits during training

It is best to completely avoid non-essential visits to the practice once the dummy run is complete. The aim will be to teach the dog first not to be worried by and then to enjoy each step of a veterinary visit. If this training is interspersed with genuinely unpleasant trips to the practice it can slow progress. The client should therefore be advised to have any necessary routine procedures performed before starting the programme and then avoid bringing their dog to the practice unless he needs non-routine medical attention. If a visit is unavoidable the possibility of using an anxiolytic medication to minimize any negative effects can be discussed with the vet.

Training at home

The owners can start by performing some of the desensitization and counter-conditioning at home. The key triggers for fearful behaviour at the vets are location and the presence of practice staff. However, the dog may also see other stimuli at the practice as predictors of something unpleasant about to happen. The effects of these triggers can be removed from the trigger stacking process (see Fig. 39) by teaching the dog not to worry about them at home.

Examples of the types of triggers and examinations the dog can learn to like at home are summarized in Box 14.9. Where equipment cannot be provided or loaned cheaply some clients may be prepared to invest in it to help their dog. The steps for teaching the dog not to be concerned by the triggers or by examinations are outlined in Box 14.10.

Teaching the dog not to worry about coming to the practice

How to teach the dog to be happy to come to the practice is outlined in Box 14.11.

The client should be advised to keep up occasional training visits to the vets even after the programme is complete to keep the positive associations strong in case of future unavoidably unpleasant visits.

Fireworks and storms

Many dogs are fearful of fireworks and storms. In some cases this may spread to a more generalized sound sensitivity. The flow chart in Appendix 13 identifies those cases where the fear is more severe or generalized and so requires referral to an accredited behaviourist. Other cases in which the dog's fear is limited to these very specific triggers may be suited to being treated at home using desensitization and counter-conditioning under the guidance of the practice team.

How does it work?

Desensitization is a process whereby the dog learns not to be afraid of gradually louder noises by being exposed to them in such a calm and safe way that he stops paying attention to them. Counter-conditioning is the process of linking the sounds with a more pleasant emotion such as pleasure linked to food, play or fuss. Desensitization is required before counter-conditioning as any fear the dog feels will prevent the dog getting pleasure from the food, etc. Counter-conditioning is needed after desensitization because desensitization can break down very easily with one unpleasant experience such as a particularly loud bang. Counter-conditioning protects against this. These principles are discussed more in Chapter 7.

When to start

The dog's exposure to the trigger sounds needs to be controlled throughout the training period. It is therefore important to take steps to avoid the dog being exposed to any real sounds during the same period as he is undergoing desensitization and counter-conditioning. This will ensure he is not exposed to sounds that are louder than he has so far learned to accept.

For fear of fireworks this is best achieved by starting at a time of year when there are least likely to be real fireworks. As these are typically associated with celebrations and festivals they tend to be

Box 14.9. Triggers, equipment and examinations the client can train their dog to accept at home.

- Smells, e.g. skin antiseptics, environmental disinfectants and spirit.
- Veterinary uniforms.
- Visually examining various body parts, e.g. ears, teeth, eyes, paws, tummy and under the tail. Name each body part as doing so (see Table 42, Chapter 10).
- Touching the dog wearing examination gloves.
- Syringes and needles being placed close to the dogs scruff and foreleg.

- Using a stethoscope to listen to a dog's chest or abdomen.
- Placing an auroscope/otoscope specula in the ear (as long as there is no inflammation or pain).
- Using a penlight torch for eye examination.
- Opening and closing nail clippers close to the toes.
- Switching electric clippers on and off and holding close to the dogs foreleg.

Box 14.10. Desensitizing and counter-conditioning a dog to practice triggers, equipment and examinations.

- The trigger/equipment should be placed on a work surface or table where the dog can see it. The dog should be allowed to withdraw if he wants to.
- Advise the client to observe for signs of stress and increase the distance between the trigger and the dog if any are seen. If they persist when the trigger is placed as far away as it can be the client should be referred to an accredited behaviourist.
- The client should perform some reward-based training, play a game or give the dog some treats. Once the training or game is over the trigger is put away again.

- This should be repeated until the dog looks excited when the trigger is brought out.
- The trigger can then be brought slightly closer and the above steps repeated until the dog again looks happy when the trigger is brought out.
- The trigger should continue to be gradually brought closer step by step until the dog is happy for the trigger to be next to him or to be touched with it. The dog should be completely happy at one distance before proceeding to the next. This will take multiple sessions.
- The client should then start to perform examinations with the equipment using the step by step principles above.

---

quite predictable. However, ensure the client considers the range of cultural festivals that use fireworks for celebration, not just those they celebrate themselves. Common festivals that are often celebrated with fireworks are summarized in Box 14.12. The aim for storm phobias is to choose the time of year when storms are least likely to occur.

Management strategies

As training cannot always be started straight away clients may need to be advised how to manage their dog's fear of sounds in the interim. Strategies for doing so are summarized in Box 14.13 and discussed below.

Adaptil™ is a synthetic version of a canine calming pheromone. There is extensive evidence to suggest it can help reduce fear and anxiety in situations such as this. Use of a diffuser or collar is therefore recommended during firework and storm seasons. The mode and effect of use is discussed in Chapter 7. The diffuser or collar should be started 1–2 two weeks before the anticipated noise season and continued for 1 week after.

Providing a den (escape to safety) can ensure the dog feels he has a place to retreat to when feeling concerned. Key principles for den design are discussed in Chapter 7. Dens used in sound-sensitive dogs need to be positioned away from windows and doors and benefit from additional sound insulation such as foam or blankets over the top. Layered blankets inside the den also enable the dog

Box 14.11. Desensitizing and counter-conditioning a dog to visiting the practice.

- The dog should be taken to the point immediately before the point at which he first looked worried on the dummy run.
- The client should stand quietly and allow the dog to take in his environment. This is the desensitization process. If the client sees any signs of fear or stress they should go back a step and try again.
- Once the dog starts to look bored or disinterested they should perform some reward-based training, give the dog some treats, play a game or fuss the dog to make it a pleasurable experience. This is the counter-conditioning.
- They should continue for about 10 min then end the session.
- This step should be repeated until the dog looks excited when he arrives. The client can then progress to the next step, e.g. move from the car park to the front door.
- The process should be repeated until the dog is again excited as soon as he arrives. They can then move on to the next step.

- Each step should be gone through in turn until the dog can enter the consulting room and be put on the table without concern.
- If the dog is making rapid progress it may be possible to progress immediately to a subsequent step without needing to go back another day. However, desensitization and counter-conditioning to the veterinary practice is very likely to be challenged by a negative experience at some stage. Taking time to establish repeated strong positive links along the way is the best protection against this. This will take multiple sessions.
- If at any time the dog shows fear or stress the client should go home, start again at an earlier step next time and proceed more slowly. It is common to have odd 'off' days.
- If the dog is showing stress at even the very first sign of going to the vets or not making any progress, refer the client to an accredited behaviourist.

Box 14.12. Festivals or events that are commonly celebrated with fireworks.

- Guy Fawkes night.
- New Year's Eve.
- Chinese New Year.
- Diwali.
- 4th July.
- Jubilees, royal weddings etc.
- Presidential inaugurations.

The dog should be taken out for exercise and elimination before the trigger sounds start. Other stimuli the dog may find distressing should be avoided, e.g. if the dog is bothered by the vacuum cleaner the client should avoid using it after dark or during storms.

Curtains should be closed and toys or treats made available to distract the dog with. Music, especially something with a rhythmic beat, can help mask sound, as can the TV or white noise, e.g. a fan.

The client should stay with the dog, but show no reaction to the sounds. They should avoid fussing over the dog as this may send the message there is something to be afraid of or teach him to show fear to get attention. Equally he should not be ignored or he may start to associate the sounds with the punishment of being ignored. The client should just try to behave as normally as possible. If the dog becomes fearful and is unable to settle himself he may be able to be distracted by playing a game or doing some training, although he should not be forced.

Anxiolytic medication such as benzodiazepines may be indicated in extreme cases.

The sound recording

There are many sound recordings available designed for use in sound desensitization and

to hide under them. When using added insulation and blankets ensure there is sufficient air circulation to prevent overheating. Never confine the dog in the den. If there is no room for a den or the dog does not take to it, ensure the room the dog will be in during firework displays or storms will absorb sound. Rooms with soft furnishings, carpets and covered windows are far preferable to rooms with hard floors, large or uncovered windows or large expanses of hard surfaces, such as kitchens, conservatories or utility rooms. The dog's normal sleeping place may need to be temporarily changed to accommodate this.

> **Box 14.13. Management strategies for sound phobias.**
>
> - Adaptil™ diffuser or collar.
> - A soundproof den.
> - Exercise before noises start.
> - Avoiding any other triggers the dog is worried by, e.g. vacuum cleaner.
> - Staying with the dog.
>
> - Stay calm. Neither fuss or ignore.
> - Closing curtains.
> - Using white noise or music with a rhythmic beat.
> - Anxiolytic medication such as benzodiazepines may be indicated in some cases.

counter-conditioning. Some are more effective than others. The key criteria for choosing a sound recording is that it is long enough and variable enough to not become too predictable or repetitive so the dog does not learn to accept that pattern of sound but not variations from it. It is also important that the recording includes numerous sudden sounds with long gaps in between, as this is the type of sound that causes the greatest reaction. It is therefore essential that these are part of the programme. The sound quality of the recording is also important to success.

The CD needs to be tested to ensure the individual dog reacts to it in the same way as he does to real sounds before use, as if he does not then the process will be ineffective. The CD should be initially set up and tested whilst the dog is out – perhaps on a walk. Responses are generally better if the sound comes from somewhere unpredictable. Many dogs have learned to ignore sound that comes from the household CD or DVD player. It is therefore better to use a good quality portable sound system such as a portable CD player, mobile phone or mp3 player that can be moved around. The player should initially be set up in the room the dog will normally be in or go to when the sounds naturally occur. Speakers placed by a window or door and obscured from view add realism. Bass and treble should be adjusted to make the sounds as realistic as possible and any special effects switched off.

The next step is to test the dog's reactions to the sound recordings. The client should choose the track that provokes the strongest response in their dog, e.g. if he is most bothered by banging fireworks use recordings of this for the test. He or she should start the recording at the lowest volume and gradually increase this over approximately 1 min. As soon as the dog shows any signs of stress to the noise the test can be stopped. The client should then make a

note of the signs their particular dog shows. If the dog does not react at all even at full volume the recording will not work. However, it is worthwhile trying other recordings due to variations in quality.

Teaching the dog not to be concerned by the noises

Where a CD or album has multiple recordings, start with the one that is likely to provoke the least intense response for the dog. For example, if a CD has recordings of firework whistles and bangs and the dog is most concerned by bangs then start the training with the recording of whistles. Expose the dog to this recording at the lowest volume setting and gradually increase its intensity as outlined in Box 14.14.

It is important the client acts as if nothing unusual is going on during the training. Giving extra attention may signal to the dog there is something to be afraid of or may teach the dog to use fearful body language to get attention. Equally, ignoring the dog is a punishment and so ignoring him completely may strengthen the link between the sounds and unpleasant sensations. The client should act as if there is nothing unusual happening. It may also help to provide an Adaptil™ diffuser or collar and a soundproof den during training, as discussed in management above.

At least some of the training should be performed after dark for firework phobia as the dog will associate darkness with fireworks. Once the programme is complete it will make the conditioning stronger if the recordings are also played in different rooms and outside such as in the garden or in the car. This should be started again at lower levels and gradually increase as before. Progress during these subsequent stages is usually much faster than in the first stage of training.

Box 14.14. Teaching a dog not to be concerned by noises.

- The volume should be set to zero and the CD started.
- The volume should then be gradually increased until the dog's behaviour indicates he can hear the sounds (e.g. ear twitching or interest) but is not showing any of signs of fear or stress. If he looks worried the volume should be reduced again until he stops.
- The recording should be played for about 15 min, two or three times a day, whilst the owner goes about their normal activities. The door to the room with the speakers in should be left open so the dog can leave if he wants to.
- This should be repeated every day until the dog is not reacting at all. The owner can then start to play with the dog or perform some treat training whilst the CD is playing to counter-condition him to it. This should be repeated twice a day until he looks excited when the noise comes on.
- Increase the volume very slightly and repeat.
- This process is repeated until the dog is happy to play or train at the highest volume the dog will experience during a real firework event or storm.
- The process is then repeated for the different tracks on the CD, ending with the track combining sudden noises with long gaps.
- If at any stage the dog starts to show signs of fear or stress the CD should be stopped and restarted another day using a lower setting.
- If the dog is strongly fearful or distressed at even the lowest setting the client can try switching off one speaker, muffling the speaker with a cushion or moving the stereo to another room. If he is still concerned after these modifications the client should be referred to an accredited behaviourist.

15 Making a Referral

The practice has a professional responsibility to ensure that any referrals they make are to suitably qualified and accredited professionals. There is currently no statutory regulation of the dog training and behaviour modification industry either in the UK or the USA. As such anyone can proclaim themselves to be a trainer or behaviourist. This leads to enormous variation in the abilities and techniques used. As discussed in Chapter 7, some methods compromise animal welfare and can be potentially harmful. Failure to correct behaviour can have equally detrimental long-term results if it leads to relinquishment or euthanasia. Care must therefore be taken when choosing to whom to make the referral. The following assumes the practice does not have an in-house behavioural specialist.

Trainer or Behaviourist?

The first consideration is whether the dog requires the advice of a trainer or a behaviourist. Although there is considerable cross-over between the two, they are not the same.

Trainer

Dog trainers primarily offer services that show clients how to manage their dog's everyday behaviour using operant conditioning (see Chapter 7). This will usually involve teaching basic commands and good manners. The types of behaviours the American College of Veterinary Behaviourists (ACVB) suggest fall to a trainer are summarized in Box 15.1. Precisely which of these services an individual trainer offers will depend on their training, experience and preference. Many will also offer classes in teaching sports or tricks (see Chapter 7).

Evaluating a trainer

There is no recognized route to qualify as a dog trainer. Some may have followed a formal course of study of variable quality. Others may have learned through a less structured route ranging from being mentored by an accredited trainer to being entirely self-taught from books, online resources, TV programmes and maybe even trial and error with their own dogs. As there is no one recognized or correct route the only way to know if a trainer is someone the practice can reliably refer to is to determine to what degree they have the theoretical understanding and practical experience needed to be competent.

The practice can research a trainer's abilities themselves. Table 57 and Box 15.2 outline the theoretical knowledge, practical experience and other considerations they should take into account when doing so. It is recommended that someone from the practice personally observes a class and talks to the trainer afterwards rather than relying on recommendations, unless from another accredited trainer or behaviourist.

Dog training accreditation bodies

There are a number of bodies that offer to accredit dog trainers as competent. These may offer the practice a simpler way of identifying trainers to which they can confidently send clients. However, there is no regulation of these bodies and their requirements for accreditation are very variable. The practice therefore needs to satisfy itself which bodies they will recognize. The factors that should be taken into consideration when doing so are summarized in Tables 58 and 59. The advantage of researching an accreditation body instead of an individual dog trainer is that once the practice has satisfied themselves that a body is reliable they can then recognize any dog trainer who is a member of it.

The behaviourist or behaviour counsellor

The term behaviourist or behaviour counsellor is generally used to refer to someone who advises how to correct or manage problem behaviour that

Box 15.1. Behaviours falling within the remit of the dog trainer (Luescher *et al.*, 2007).

- Basic management commands.
- Initial housetraining.
- Greeting behaviour, including not jumping up.
- Acceptance of veterinary examination and grooming.
- Loose lead walking.
- Preventing possessive behaviour.

- Managing and diffusing problem behaviour in the class setting.
- Correcting problem behaviour arising due to mistakes in management.
- Implementation of a programme devised by a behaviourist following diagnosis of the problem behaviour.

Table 57. Considerations when choosing a dog trainer.

Consideration	Discussion
Methods	What methods of training do they use and do they use positive punishments (see chapter 7)?
Limitations	What does the trainer do if faced with a problem they are not sure how to address? Be wary of anybody who claims this never happens.
Insurance	Are they insured?
Class size	The maximum recommended size is 8, with a staff ratio of at least 1:4, depending on ability. Assess each trainer individually. Trainer's should spend equal time with each dog.
Equipment in use	What types of collars, harnesses and other equipment is in use?
Attendees' behaviour	Observe the body language of the dogs and handlers, especially those that have been before, to see if they enjoy classes.
Advertising and websites	Verify claims made in advertising. Some make exaggerated claims or disguise their use of positive punishments.

Box 15.2. Subjects of which a dog trainer requires a theoretical knowledge.

- Canine body language and communication.
- How dogs learn.
- Techniques for teaching exercises and how these can be modified according to any special needs or characteristics of the owner or dog.
- Use of equipment.
- Welfare and stress in dogs and owners.

- Whether the dog should undergo training when suffering various health problems.
- Planning and organizing classes.
- Presentation and communication.
- Evaluation of classes.
- Business and marketing.
- Health and safety.
- Legislation.

arises for reasons other than failure to provide proper training. However, the title is not protected and so anyone can use these titles regardless of their competence to do so.

Theoretical knowledge

Behaviourists are often required to address behaviours with a complex aetiology requiring specialist treatments. They therefore need an in-depth knowledge of canine behaviour and behaviour modification techniques as well as the knowledge and skills to support the client through the process. The theoretical subjects the behaviourist needs to study are summarized in Table 60.

It would be theoretically possible for a dedicated individual to study all these subjects in sufficient depth to gain the knowledge, objectivity and evaluation skills needed for competency without following a formal course of study. However, it would be very difficult and time consuming for a practice to evaluate whether they have done so in each individual case. Therefore the only practical way for the practice to accurately assess an individual's theoretical

Table 58. Considerations when evaluating accreditation bodies.

Consideration	Discussion
Qualification requirements	Does the organization require a formal qualification? If so, the qualifications required also need to be reviewed (see Table 59).
Other membership requirements	Does the organization have any other requirements for membership or perform a formal assessment? If so, what are their assessment criteria and what are the qualifications of those performing the assessment? Do they assess practical skills?
Code of conduct	Do they have a code of conduct and if so what does it say? Look for specific guidance rather than terminology that is open to interpretation. Terms such as 'humane', 'in good faith' and 'accepted standards' are subjective and so meaningless. Exclusion of specific methods or a requirement to be able to justify methods scientifically offers greater confidence. How is adherence monitored?
Endorsements	Look for endorsement by established bodies such as humane societies (RSPCA, ASPCA etc.), veterinary bodies, recognized educational establishments or government departments.
CPD requirements	Does the association ensure members maintain knowledge and continue to develop their skills? How is this monitored?
Philosophy	What is the organization's philosophy? Look for specific guidance rather than terminology that is open to interpretation (see above).
Insurance	All accreditation bodies should require that their members carry suitable third-party and indemnity insurance.
Membership levels	Be aware that many associations have membership levels. It is important to identify not only which association the trainer or behaviourist is a member of but also at what level and any variations in the membership requirements at each level.

Table 59. Considerations when evaluating courses.

Consideration	Discussion
The education provider	Is the company recognized or accredited as an education provider? What is its reputation and standing in the education community?
The tutors	Who are the tutors and what are their own accreditations and/or qualifications?
The awarding body	Is the course formally accredited by a recognized awarding body? Does that body accredit the content or just the format of the qualification and the assessment process?
The content	Does the content cover the minimum requirements for a dog trainer or behaviourist (see Box 15.1 and Table 60)? Does the content and philosophy reflect the latest understanding of dog behaviour?
The assessment procedure	How are skills assessed? Some courses award certificates of completion based on attendance only. Others have rigorous assessment procedures that verify understanding.
The level	At what level is the qualification? The accepted level of study for a behaviourist is university graduate.

knowledge is to rely on an independently assessed academic course of study that has covered all the above subjects at the required level. See Table 59 with regard to evaluating a course of study.

Practical skills

A behaviourist also has to be competent to handle dogs safely, teach basic commands and apply practical training and behaviour modification methods. A practice can ask to observe a behaviourist doing so to assess their skills. However, unless they also run training classes (which many do), this may be challenging as the types of cases most behaviourists work with are often not suited to being observed. An alternative way to observe practical skills is to ask to see video recordings of the behaviourist's work or rely on independent accreditation (see below).

Behaviourist accreditation bodies

There are a number of bodies that offer to accredit behaviourists as competent. However, there is no regulation of them and their requirements for accreditation are very variable. The practice therefore needs

Table 60. Subjects of which a behaviourist needs a theoretical knowledge.

Subject	Comment
Species ethology	In-depth study of the behaviour of the domestic dog in its natural environment, i.e. the home. Study of wolves is not a substitute.
The physiology of behaviour	How the endocrine and nervous systems, diet, drugs and disease affect behaviour.
Influences over behaviour	In-depth study of all the influences over behaviour and how normal and abnormal behaviours develop.
Methods used to modify behaviour	Including management and manipulation of conditioning and learning, the human:dog bond, the environment and supporting therapies. They also need to be aware of physiological and pharmacological interventions that may be performed by the vet.
Human behaviour and human-animal interaction	Understanding human needs, expectations, motivations and limitations and their impact on the human:dog bond and their dog's behaviour.
Animal welfare	Understanding of the threats to an animal's welfare and the signs of suffering to ensure the dog's welfare is protected.
Counselling techniques	Methods for effective history taking, communication and on-going support and guidance, including the ethics of the role.
Law	Legislation as it applies to both the dog's behaviour and their professional conduct.

to satisfy itself which bodies they will recognize. The factors that should be taken into consideration when doing so are summarized in Tables 58 and 59. The advantage of researching an accreditation body instead of an individual behaviourist is that once the practice has satisfied themselves that a body is reliable they can then recognize any behaviourist who is a member of it.

Referral

Steps for making the referral can be agreed locally according to the practice and behaviour practitioner's preferences. Some kind of formal record is advisable for all concerned. An example referral form is given in Appendix 14.

Interim Management Advice

It may be necessary to offer interim management advice in some cases. When doing so it needs to be made clear to the client that this is purely to prevent injury or deterioration whilst the referral is being arranged and does not replace the need for behavioural assessment and treatment.

First aid

The aims of behavioural first aid are to prevent further incidents of aggression, to alleviate acute emotional distress and to temporarily manage problem behaviours to avoid injury or deterioration to such a point that the owner is no longer willing to

keep the dog. Strategies should also aim to avoid permanently changing behaviour prior to the consultation where possible, so as not to interfere with the initial diagnostic process or limit treatment options. For example, use of medication or pheromones may mask the behaviour before the behavioural specialist has had a chance to assess it. Neutering can aggravate the problem in some cases and may preclude manipulation of reproductive status where dogs that live together are fighting.

Aggression to canine or human non-family members

Inappropriate behaviour to other dogs, or to people on walks or visiting the house can be managed by ensuring the dog is under complete control whenever he in this situation. Ways to achieve this are summarized in Table 61. An aggressive dog must be in the care of a responsible adult whenever he is around other people or dogs. Such dogs must never be left in the care of a minor inside or outside of the house. Clients must be made aware of their legal liabilities should their dog injure a person or another animal

Aggression to owners

Owners should avoid behaviour known to trigger aggression. Examples of how to do so are given in Table 62. Owners should be advised not to punish the dog in any way to avoid aggravating fear or triggering the dog to escalate the level of threat being used. This includes the use of dominance/pack theory

Table 61. Immediate methods for controlling dogs showing dog or human-directed aggression to non family members.

Method	Discussion
Avoid triggers	Clients should walk in places or at times where the trigger is unlikely to be encountered. They should also be reminded owners of other dogs with issues will be doing the same so they need to give each other a wide berth.
Keep on lead	Collars or harnesses should be well fitting and in good condition. The dog should be kept on lead around triggers outside of the house.
Maintain boundaries	The client should check garden fences, gates etc. are secure to avoid escapes.
Locks	Locks should be fitted on gates to prevent people entering garden areas where the dog may be unsupervised. A wireless bell can be fitted to gates so the caller can let the client know they are there.
Muzzle	The dogs can be taught to accept a cage muzzle for use outside of the house and/or around visitors. The owner must be made aware of the increased risk this places the dog under and safety precautions for their use. This is discussed further in Appendix 4.
Exclude	If fear of or aggression to visitors is high, the dog is better excluded to prevent deterioration. If the visitor is coming to stay for a prolonged period the dog can be put in kennels or sent to stay with family or friends.

Table 62. Managing owner-directed aggression whilst awaiting a behaviour consultation.

Aggression trigger	Discussion
Toy or chew	Avoid giving the dog or allowing access to these items in the short term.
Food bowl	The dog should be fed in a separate room with the door closed. He can be released once he has finished eating and the bowls cleared away after he has left the room. Food should never be fed ad lib. Children should not be permitted to feed the dog and the dog should be excluded whilst they are eating or if they have food in their hands.
Owner's bed	Exclude the dog from the bedroom using a baby gate.
Grooming	In most cases it will not cause long-term problems if the dog is not groomed for a week or two. If it will, then sedating and clipping the coat short can avoid the need for this prior to the consultation and during the training period afterwards.
Stolen items	Clients should avoid taking things away if this triggers aggression. If the dog is at risk of injuring himself with something he has taken they can walk away scattering a trail of tasty food as they go. This lures the dog away and takes the challenge out of the situation. They can then shut the door or someone else can throw something over the item. If this does not succeed only they can make the decision between the risk of being bitten trying to remove it and leaving the item with the dog.
Approaching the dog's bed	Give the dog a place to retreat to that does not need to be approached.

or 'dog whispering' methods. See Chapter 7 for further discussion of the types of punishments people may use and the concerns associated with doing so. Clients may need to be educated in low-level threat and appeasing signals so they can read and respond to these (see Chapter 5).

Bolts or latches on interior doors, baby gates and crates can help keep dogs away from vulnerable people such as children or the elderly. However, the dog's need for exercise, stimulation and companionship must be mainlined when using these.

If the dog does threaten, the client should withdraw as outlined in Box 15.3.

Aggression between dogs in the household

If dogs are fighting over resources or in specific situations these should be temporarily eliminated. For example, fights at feeding time can be avoided by feeding in separate rooms or fights over chews can be avoided by not giving them. If the dogs are fighting on sight or the owner cannot identify the trigger they may need to be kept apart until the consultation can be arranged. In some cases alternating confinement to a crate or keeping the dogs either side of a baby gate can be sufficient to prevent fights.

Box 15.3. Withdrawal if a dog shows threat.

- Stop what they are doing.
- Keep their arms still.
- Avoid shouting or making noise other than talking calmly and quietly.
- Slowly move their body so they are at an angle to the dog.
- Put their weight on their back foot.
- Look to one side of the dog, avoiding direct eye contact.

- Move quietly and calmly away without turning their back.
- If movement escalates the level of aggression they should stop or try to move behind a solid object, e.g. a piece of furniture, a door or a gate.
- If the dog responds to control by another person that person may calmly intervene.

Others may fight through cage bars and so will need to be kept in entirely separate rooms. If the dogs do not fight on walks, which is often the case, they should continue to be walked together. If one or both dogs seem to be anxious or restless even when in entirely separate rooms it may be necessary for one dog to stay with friends or family to avoid building up greater tension or chronic stress.

Separation distress

Ideally the dog will not be left alone until the issue can be evaluated. Strategies may include short-term use of day care or dog walkers, family or friends, taking the dog in the car (weather permitting) or to work with the owner.

Further Resources

Animal Behaviour and Training Council: http://www. abtcouncil.org.uk

Association for the Study of Animal Behaviour: http:// asab.nottingham.ac.uk/accred/index.php

Association of Pet Behaviour Counsellors: http://www. apbc.org.uk

Association of Pet Dog Trainers: http://www.apdt.co.uk

Glossary

Affective aggression: Aggressive behaviour that is driven by emotion. This may be in self-defence or to defend a resource

Aggression: All elements of behaviour intended to control others through actual or the threat of harm

Agonistic: All elements of behaviour surrounding conflict

Allelomimetic: Group social behaviour such as hunting or resting

Anxiety: The expectation something unpleasant or potentially harmful will happen without any immediate indication it will

Commensal: One party to a relationship benefits without harm to the other

Conspecifics: Others of the same species

Critical period: A period of development in which the animal must undergo some experience or event for the behaviour it triggers to develop properly

Et-epimeletic: Seeking care from others

Epimeletic: Giving care to others

Ethology: The objective study of animal behaviour in the natural setting

Extinction burst: A transient increase in behaviour during operant or classical conditioning

Generalized: The spread of operant or classical conditioning to other similar situations

Habituation: The process by which an animal's emotional or behavioural response to a harmless stimulus lessens as he becomes familiar to it

Learned helplessness: Learning that no action will prevent an aversive stimulus and so no longer trying to avoid it

Mutualistic: Both parties to a relationship get equal benefit

Observational learning: Learning by observing the behaviour of others

Paedomorphosis: Retaining juvenile characteristics

Parasitic: One party in a relationship benefits at the expense of the other

Phenotype: The physiology and morphology of an individual

Progenitor: The animal's ancestral species

Appendix 1

Poster promoting the principle of using a yellow ribbon to indicate a dog that does not like being approached (© Yellow Dog UK. Copies available at: http://www.yellowdoguk.co.uk).

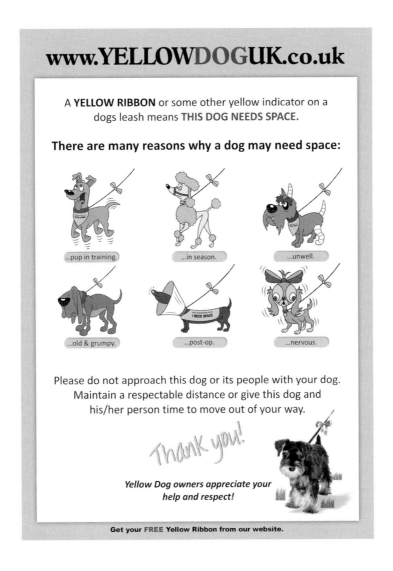

Appendix 2

Advice poster for handling stressed dogs in practice by APBC (© APBC. Copies available at: http://www.apbc.org.uk).

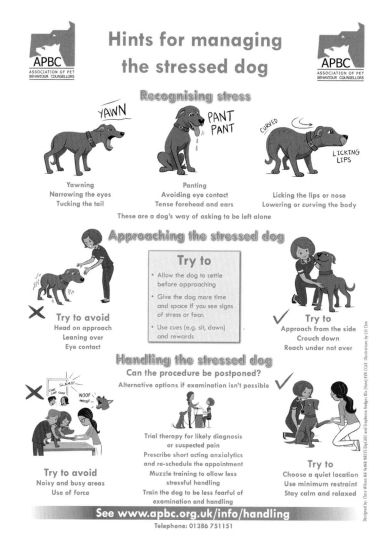

Appendix 3
Example Patient Behaviour Assessment

Collating the following information about a dog's behaviour can help practice staff ensure the dog's triggers are controlled and so lower the risk the dog may use aggression, using the trigger stacking principle.

1. Does your dog approach and greet people happily?
2. Does your dog approach and greet other dogs happily?
3. Is your dog worried by noises, people or dogs?
4. Does your dog tend to turn his back on people or dogs?
5. Does your dog lower his head, look away, cower or run away from anything? If so please give details.
6. Has your dog ever growled or curled his lip at you, a visitor or person outside of the vets?
7. Does your dog ever seem worried by coming to the vets?
8. Are there any parts of the body your dog does like being touched on? If so, what does he do?
9. Has your dog had a stay in hospital before? If so, how did the staff say he coped?
10. Has the dog ever growled or lunged at another dog? If so, does this happen occasionally or often?
11. Is your dog used to a crate and if so how does he respond if people approach him when he is in it?
12. Is your dog happy to be touched by the collar?
13. Has the dog ever injured anyone or another dog?
14. Has anyone ever said they felt afraid of your dog?
15. Is your dog happy on an examination table?
16. How does your dog respond to injections?
17. Does your dog show fear of anything? If so, please give details.
18. Is your dog bothered by cats or other pet species?
19. What are your dog's favourite treats or games?
20. Is your dog familiar with wearing a muzzle?

Where responses to questions indicate the dog may be showing problem behaviour ask for clarification and discuss options for correcting this behaviour. Aim to ask questions in a relaxed and non-judgemental manner.

Appendix 4
Client Fact Sheet

Teaching a Dog to Wear a Cage Muzzle

1. Identify the signs your dog shows when he is worried by something. These can include cowering, tucking his tail, putting his ears back, trying to escape, shaking, whining, growling, yawning or licking his lips.

2. Place the muzzle somewhere your dog can see it but not reach it and leave it there for about 15 min. Make sure your dog can get away from the muzzle if he feels the need, e.g. go into another room. Carry on as if nothing is happening. Neither give extra attention nor ignore your dog. Repeat 3/4 times a day until he shows none of the signs of distress identified above on two successive training sessions, then move on to the next step.

3. Hold the muzzle near to your dog, give him a treat and then hide the muzzle behind your back. Repeat four or five times. Make sure he can get away from it if he wants. Repeat as above until he is ready for the next step.

4. Hold the muzzle in your hand and place a food treat just inside. Let your dog take it. It is important he chooses to put his nose in to take the treat rather than the muzzle being pushed on to his nose. Repeat four or five times. If he tries to take the treat any other way just ignore it. Repeat as above until he is ready for the next step.

5. Place the treat in the muzzle and allow your dog to take it as above. Fiddle with the muzzle straps and touch the back of your dog's neck as he takes the treat. Repeat as above until he is ready for the next step.

6. Smear a soft foodstuff such as peanut butter or cream cheese inside the front of the muzzle and allow your dog to lick it. As he does so clip the straps closed loosely. Allow him to finish licking the food stuff then remove the muzzle. Repeat as above.

7. Smear the inside of the front of the muzzle with a soft foodstuff and clip the strap together so it fits correctly. Allow him to finish licking the food stuff and then leave the muzzle on for a few more minutes then remove. Repeat as above.

8. Once your dog is wearing the muzzle happily start to put it on for a few minutes randomly at times when he is distracted, e.g. on a walk. Maintain doing so even when he is no longer worried by it so it is not a sign of something stressful.

The speed of progress will vary between dogs. It is important that you only move to a later step once your dog is clearly relaxed with the current one.

When using the muzzle bear in mind the following precautions:

- A muzzle only reduces the possibility for injury. Dogs can still cause minor teeth injuries, bruising, scratching or emotional distress and no muzzle is indestructible. Do not feed your dog whilst wearing the muzzle other than small training treats.

- Do not leave your dog unattended with the muzzle on. He could choke if he vomits or he tries to scavenge food whilst wearing the muzzle.

- Your dog is at risk if attacked by another dog when wearing the muzzle, so prevent or provide close supervision of all interactions with other dogs.

Appendix 5
Example Socialization and Habituation Record Chart

Experience	8 weeks	9 weeks	10 weeks	11 weeks	12 weeks
Men					
Women					
Babies					
Preschool children					
School children					
Teenagers					
Elderly people					
Physically disabled people					
People with different skin colours					
People in uniforms					
People wearing hats/crash helmets					
People carrying sticks					
Approach of delivery people					
House visitors					
Other dogs					
Other puppies					
Cats					
Rabbits					
Captive birds					
Horses					
Livestock					
Car rides					
Bus or train rides					
Bicycles					
Busy towns					
Countryside					
Parks					
Grooming with a soft brush					
Examining all over body					
Escalators and lifts					
Washing machine					
TV					
Lawn mower					
Vacuum cleaner					
Thunder, fireworks, gunshot					
Cuddling and handling head and neck					

Appendix 6
Client Fact Sheet

Introducing Basic Puppy Commands

The following provides guidance in the very first steps in teaching puppy commands. This can then be built on through training classes as the puppy develops. When training puppies keep in mind:

- At this age puppies have very short attention spans and so will be easily distracted. Keep training bouts short and fun. Only practise one command at a time and have a break before trying another one.
- Also match the command word to spontaneously performed behaviours and then reward them.
- If your puppy is bored or not able to focus, try again later.
- Ignore failures – just try again next time. Never punish or get angry with your puppy – he just has not yet learnt what you want him to do.
- Choose rewards that work for your puppy. This can include fuss, play, toys and treats. Keeping special toys for training makes them more rewarding. Treats should be small and non-fattening. If your puppy is happy to work for his kibble this is great, but if he is not excited by it you may need to use something else.

Sit

- Lure your puppy to sit by passing a treat backwards 15 cm above his head.
- As your puppy's bottom touches the ground say 'sit' and give him the treat.
- Repeat four or five times, two or three times a day.

Stay

- Ask your puppy to sit.
- As long as your puppy is sitting still say 'stay' and give a treat.
- Repeat four or five times, then use a jolly voice to release him.

- Repeat two or three times a day.
- When your puppy is starting to find this easy you can start to very gradually move away, starting by just rocking on to your back foot and building up to taking one step away.

Give

- Give your puppy a moderately desirable toy.
- Once he is engaged with it show your puppy a treat and wait for your puppy to drop the toy so he can take the treat.
- As he does so say the word 'give', then allow him to take the treat.
- Once he has eaten the treat give him back the toy.
- Repeat four or five times, two or three times a day.

Leave

- Place a treat approximately 20 cm in front of your puppy.
- Hold your hand over the treat and keep it there until the puppy stops trying to steal it.
- Slowly move your hand away. Say 'leave' as you do so.
- If your puppy tries to steal the treat cover it over again and repeat.
- If he does not try to steal it for 1 s give it to him.
- Repeat four or five times, two or three times a day.

Recall

- Hold a treat in front of your puppy and walk slowly backwards, far enough that your puppy has to take four or five paces to reach you.
- As your puppy follows, you say 'come'.
- When he reaches you give him a treat.
- Repeat four or five times, two or three times a day.

 Practical Canine Behaviour: For Veterinary Nurses and Technicians (S. Hedges)

Appendix 7
When to Refer: Elimination in the house

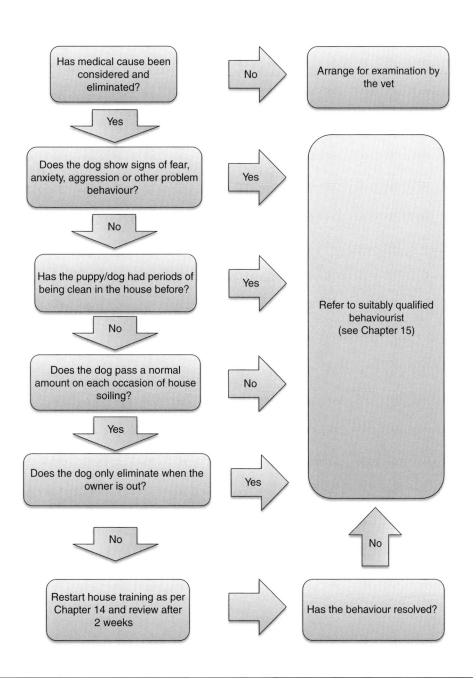

Has medical cause been considered and eliminated?

No → Arrange for examination by the vet

Yes ↓

Does the dog show signs of fear, anxiety, aggression or other problem behaviour?

Yes →

No ↓

Has the puppy/dog had periods of being clean in the house before?

Yes →

No ↓

Does the dog pass a normal amount on each occasion of house soiling?

No →

Yes ↓

Does the dog only eliminate when the owner is out?

Yes →

No ↓

Restart house training as per Chapter 14 and review after 2 weeks

→ Has the behaviour resolved?

No ↑

Refer to suitably qualified behaviourist (see Chapter 15)

Appendix 8
When to Refer: Jumping up and mouthing

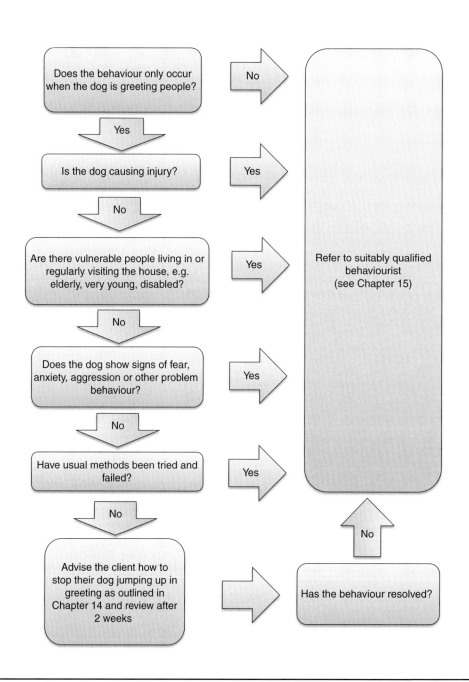

© S. Hedges 2014. *Practical Canine Behaviour: For Veterinary Nurses and Technicians* (S. Hedges)

Appendix 9
Client Fact Sheet

Teaching an Older Dog not to Jump Up During Greeting

- Ask your dog to sit when greeting.
- If your dog responds by sitting, crouch down to eye level and greet him warmly. People who are unable to crouch down to the dog's level can sit down.
- If the dog jumps up completely ignore him. Do not look at him or tell him off and avoid pushing him away as this can be interpreted as attention or even play and so may inadvertently encourage the behaviour. Turning your back often repels the dog without paying attention.
- If he is persistent leave the room without comment. Wait for 1–2 min then try again. Your leaving the room is preferable to trying to put your dog out of the room as it prevents paying him attention as you do so.

Appendix 10
When to Refer: Stealing

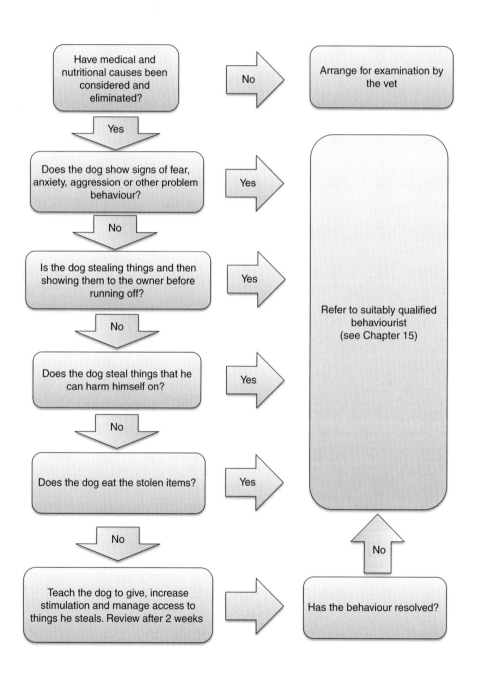

Have medical and nutritional causes been considered and eliminated? — No → Arrange for examination by the vet

Yes ↓

Does the dog show signs of fear, anxiety, aggression or other problem behaviour? — Yes →

No ↓

Is the dog stealing things and then showing them to the owner before running off? — Yes →

No ↓

Does the dog steal things that he can harm himself on? — Yes →

No ↓

Does the dog eat the stolen items? — Yes →

Refer to suitably qualified behaviourist (see Chapter 15)

No ↓

Teach the dog to give, increase stimulation and manage access to things he steals. Review after 2 weeks → Has the behaviour resolved? — No ↑

Appendix 11
When to Refer: Destructiveness and chewing

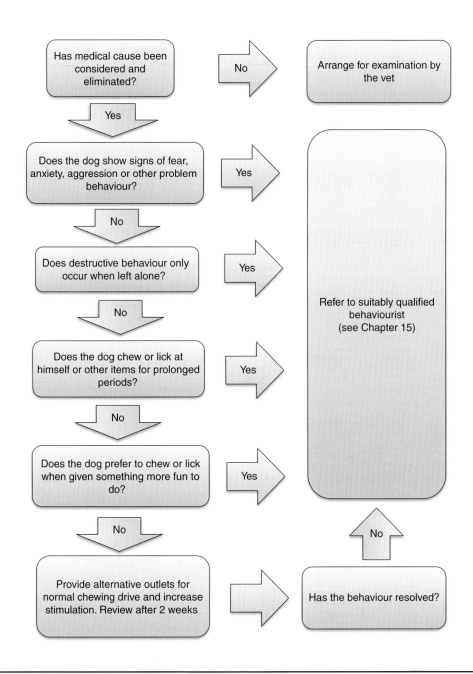

Has medical cause been considered and eliminated? → **No** → Arrange for examination by the vet

↓ **Yes**

Does the dog show signs of fear, anxiety, aggression or other problem behaviour? → **Yes** → Refer to suitably qualified behaviourist (see Chapter 15)

↓ **No**

Does destructive behaviour only occur when left alone? → **Yes** → Refer to suitably qualified behaviourist (see Chapter 15)

↓ **No**

Does the dog chew or lick at himself or other items for prolonged periods? → **Yes** → Refer to suitably qualified behaviourist (see Chapter 15)

↓ **No**

Does the dog prefer to chew or lick when given something more fun to do? → **Yes** → Refer to suitably qualified behaviourist (see Chapter 15)

↓ **No**

Provide alternative outlets for normal chewing drive and increase stimulation. Review after 2 weeks → Has the behaviour resolved?

Has the behaviour resolved? → **No** ↑ → Refer to suitably qualified behaviourist (see Chapter 15)

Appendix 12
When to Refer: Coprophagy

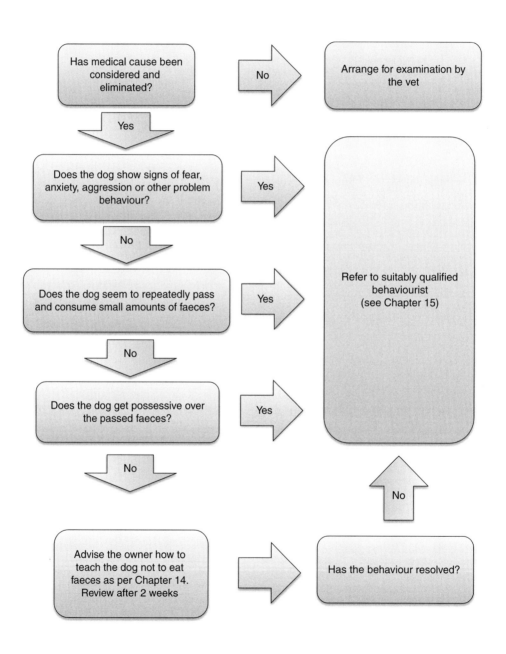

Has medical cause been considered and eliminated?

No → Arrange for examination by the vet

Yes ↓

Does the dog show signs of fear, anxiety, aggression or other problem behaviour?

Yes →

No ↓

Does the dog seem to repeatedly pass and consume small amounts of faeces?

Yes →

No ↓

Does the dog get possessive over the passed faeces?

Yes →

Refer to suitably qualified behaviourist (see Chapter 15)

No ↓

Advise the owner how to teach the dog not to eat faeces as per Chapter 14. Review after 2 weeks

→ Has the behaviour resolved?

No ↑

Appendix 13
When to Refer: Noise phobia

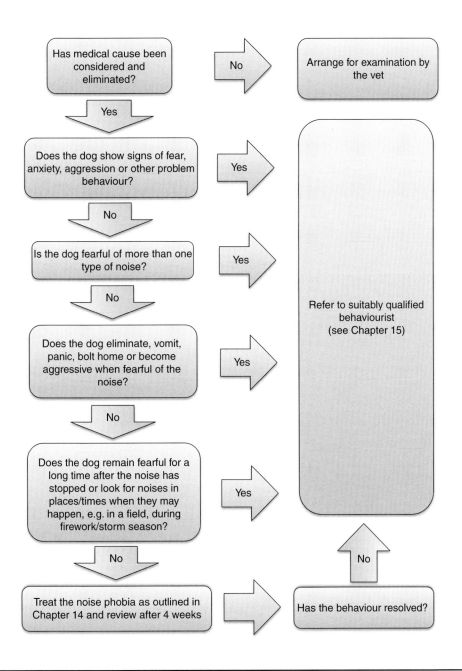

Has medical cause been considered and eliminated? → No → Arrange for examination by the vet

↓ Yes

Does the dog show signs of fear, anxiety, aggression or other problem behaviour? → Yes → Refer to suitably qualified behaviourist (see Chapter 15)

↓ No

Is the dog fearful of more than one type of noise? → Yes → Refer to suitably qualified behaviourist (see Chapter 15)

↓ No

Does the dog eliminate, vomit, panic, bolt home or become aggressive when fearful of the noise? → Yes → Refer to suitably qualified behaviourist (see Chapter 15)

↓ No

Does the dog remain fearful for a long time after the noise has stopped or look for noises in places/times when they may happen, e.g. in a field, during firework/storm season? → Yes → Refer to suitably qualified behaviourist (see Chapter 15)

↓ No

Treat the noise phobia as outlined in Chapter 14 and review after 4 weeks → Has the behaviour resolved? → No ↑ Refer to suitably qualified behaviourist

Appendix 14
Example Referral Form

Behaviour problems may arise both directly and indirectly as a result of concurrent or previous medical problems. Veterinary involvement is therefore essential in eliminating organic causes of the problem and prioritizing the diagnostic and treatment strategy to be used in any given case. In order to safeguard the welfare of your patient and indicate your approval of referral, please complete the following form.

Referring Veterinary Surgeon _____ MRCVS

Practice name

Practice address

Practice email (if appropriate)

Client name   Patient name

Client address

Client phone no.

Brief details of behaviour problem including date first noticed_____

_____

Has euthanasia been considered? Yes/No

I hereby refer the above named client to _____ for behaviour management.

Signed _____ Date _____

Please attach a full clinical history

References

Arhant, C., Bubna-Littitz, H., Bartels, A., Futschik, A. and Troxler, J. (2010) Behaviour of smaller and larger dogs: effects of training methods, inconsistency of owner behaviour and level of engagement in activities with the dog. *Applied Animal Behaviour Science* 123, 131–142.

Axelsson, E., Ratnakumar, A., Arendt, M., Maqbool, K., Webster, M.T., Perloski, M., Liberg, O., Arnemo, J.M., Hedhammar, A. and Lindblad-Toh, K. (2013) The genomic signature of dog domestication reveals adaptation to a starch-rich diet. *Nature* 495, 360–364.

Beaver, B.V. (1983) Clinical classification of canine aggression. *Applied Animal Ethology* 10, 35–43.

Bernhard, R., Rakowitz, S. and Eure, J. (2009) Immediate and Cumulative Benefits from Tellington TTouch Program Reflected in the EEG of An Anxious Mare. Available at: http://www.ttouch.com/PDFs/BenefitsTTouchEEG.pdf (accessed 27 August 2013).

Blackwell, E.J., Bolster, C., Richards, G., Loftus, B.A. and Casey, R.A. (2012) The use of electronic collars for training domestic dogs: estimated prevalence, reasons and risk factors for use, and owner perceived success as compared to other training methods. *BMC Veterinary Research* 8, 93.

Bollen, K.S. and Horowitz, J. (2008) Behavioral evaluation and demographic information in the assessment of aggressiveness in shelter dogs. *Applied Animal Behaviour Science* 112(1–2), 120–135.

Bradshaw, J.W.S., Blackwell, E.J. and Casey, R.A. (2009) Dominance in domestic dogs: useful construct or bad habit? *Journal of Veterinary Behavior* 4, 135–144.

Cavanagh, J.F., Frank, M.J. and Allen, J.J.B. (2011) Social stress reactivity alters reward and punishment learning. *Social Cognitive and Affective Neuroscience* 6, 311–320.

Cooper, J., Cracknell, N., Hardiman, J. and Mills, D. (2013a) *Studies to assess the effects of pet training aids, specifically remote static pulse systems, on the welfare of domestic dogs; field study of dogs in training.* Final report on DEFRA Project AW1402A. University of Lincoln and University of Bristol.

Cooper, J., Wright, H., Mills, D., Casey, R., Blackwell, E., van Driel, K. and Lines, J. (2013b) *Studies to assess the effects of pet training aids, specifically remote static pulse systems, on the welfare of domestic dogs.* University of Lincoln and University of Bristol.

Cottam, N., Dodman, N. and Hab, J.C. (2013) The effectiveness of the Anxiety Wrap in the treatment of canine thunderstorm phobia: an open-label trial. *Journal of Veterinary Behavior* 8, 154–161.

Deputte, B.L. and Doll, A. (2011) Do dogs understand human facial expressions? *Journal of Veterinary Behavior* 6(1), 78.

Donaldson, J. (1996) *The Culture Clash.* James & Kenneth, Oakville, Ontario.

Elliot, O. and Scott, J.P. (1961) The development of emotional stress reactions to separation in puppies. *Journal Genetic Psychology* 99, 3–22.

Farago, T., Pongracz, P., Range, F., Viranyi, Z. and Miklosi, A. (2010) 'The bone is mine': affective and referential aspects of dog growls. *Animal Behaviour* 79, 917–925.

Frank, D., Minero, M., Cannas, S. and Palestrini, C. (2007) Puppy behaviours when left home alone: a pilot study. *Applied Animal Behaviour Science* 104, 61–70.

Galton, F. (1863) *The First Steps Towards Domestication of Animals.* Spottiswoode & Co., London.

Gazzano, A., Mariti, C., Alvares, S., Cozzi, A., Tognetti, R. and Sighieri, C. (2008) The prevention of undesirable behaviors in dogs: effectiveness of veterinary behaviorists' advice given to puppy owners. *Journal of Veterinary Behavior* 3, 125–133.

Grandin, T. (1992) Calming effects of deep touch pressure in patients with autistic disorder, college students, and animals. *Journal of Child and Adolescent Psychopharmacology* 2, 1.

Grohmann, K., Dickomeit, M.J., Schmidt, M.J. and Kramer, M. (2013) Severe brain damage after punitive training technique with a choke chain collar in a German shepherd dog. *Journal of Veterinary Behavior* 8, 180–184.

Guo, K., Meints, K., Hall, C., Hall, S. and Mills, D. (2009) Left gaze bias in humans, rhesus monkeys and domestic dogs. *Animal Cognition* 12(3), 409–418.

Hecht, J., Miklósi, A. and Gácsi, M. (2012) Behavioral assessment and owner perceptions of behaviors associated with guilt in dogs. *Applied Animal Behaviour Science* 139, 134–142.

Herron, M., Shofer, F.S. and Reisner, L.R. (2009) Survey of the use and outcome of confrontational and non-confrontational training methods in client-owned dogs showing undesired behaviors. *Applied Animal Behaviour Science* 117, 47–54.

Hiby, E.J., Rooney, N.J. and Bradshaw, J.W.S. (2004) Dog training methods: their use, effectiveness and interaction with behaviour and welfare. *Animal Welfare* 13, 63–69.

Hodgetts, S. (2010) Behavioural and Physiological Effects of Weighted Vests for Children with Autism. PhD Thesis., The University of Alberta, Canada.

Hodgetts, S., Magill-Evans, J. and Misiaszek, J.E. (2011) Weighted vests, stereotyped behaviors and arousal in children with autism. *Journal of Autism and Developmental Disorders* 41(6), 805–814.

Horowitz, A. (2009) Disambiguating the 'guilty look': salient prompts to a familiar dog behaviour. *Behavioural Processes* 81, 447–452.

Houpt, K.A. and Smith, S.L. (1981) Taste preferences and their relation to obesity in dogs and cats. *The Canadian Veterinary Journal* 22(4), 77–81.

Knol, B.W. (1987) Behavioural problems in dogs. *Veterinary Quarterly* 9(3), 226–234.

Kubinyi, E., Topal, J., Miklósi, A. and Csányi, V. (2003) Dogs (*Canis familiaris*) learn from their owners via observation in a manipulation task. *Journal of Comparative Psychology* 117(2), 156–165.

Luescher, A.U., Flannigan, G. and Mertens, P. (2007) The role and limitations of trainers in behaviour treatment and therapy. *Journal of Veterinary Behaviour: Clinical Applications and Research* 2, 26–27.

Mader, B. and Hart, L.A. (1992) Establishing a model pet loss support hotline. *Journal of the American Veterinary Medical Association* 200, 270–274.

McCann, D., Barrett, A., Cooper, A., Crumpler, D., Dalen, L., Grimshaw, K., Kitchin, E., Lok, K., Porteous, L., Prince, E., Sonuga-Barke, E., Warner, J. and Stevenson, J. (2007) Food additives and hyperactive behaviour in 3-year-old and 8/9-year-old children in the community: a randomised, double-blinded, placebo-controlled trial. *Lancet* 370, 1560–1566.

Miklósi, A., Kubinyi, E., Topal, J., Gácsi, M., Viranyi, Z. and Csányi, V. (2003) A simple reason for a big difference: wolves do not look back at humans, but Dogs Do. *Current Biology* 13, 763–766.

Miller, D.D., Staats, S.R., Partlo, C. and Rada, K. (1996) Factors associated with the decision to surrender a pet to an animal shelter. *Journal of the American Veterinary Medical Association* 209, 738–742.

Miller, P.E. and Murphy, C.J. (1995) Vision in dogs. *Journal of the American Veterinary Medical Association* 207(12), 1623–1634.

Mills, D.S., Ramos, D., Estelles, M.G. and Hargrave, C. (2006) A triple blind placebo-controlled investigation into the assessment of the effect of Dog Appeasing Pheromone (DAP) on anxiety related behaviour of problem dogs in the veterinary clinic. *Applied Animal Behaviour Science* 98, 114–126.

Mills, D.S., Braem Dube, M. and Zulch, H. (2012) *Stress and Pheromonatherapy in Small Animal Clinical Behaviour*. John Wiley & Sons, Chichester, UK.

Mongillo, P., Bono, G., Regolin, L. and Marinelli, L. (2010) Selective attention to humans in companion dogs, *Canis familiaris*. *Animal Behaviour* 80, 1057–1063.

Notari, L. and Mills, D. (2011) Possible behavioral effects of exogenous corticosteroids on dog behavior: a preliminary investigation. *Journal of Veterinary Behavior: Clinical Applications and Research* 6(6), 321–327.

Olsen, P.N., Husted, P.W., Allen, T.A. and Nett, T.M. (1984) Reproductive endocrinology and physiology of the bitch and queen. *Veterinary Clinics of North America Small Animal Practice* 14, 927–946.

O'Neill, D.G., Church, D.B., McGreevy, P.D., Thomson, P.C. and Brodbelt, D.C. (2013) Longevity and mortality of owned dogs in England. *The Veterinary Journal* 198(3), 638–643.

Overall, K.L. (2003) Medical differentials with potential behavioural manifestations. *Clinical Techniques in Small Animal Practice* 19(4), 250–258.

Pongracz, P., Molnar, C. and Miklósi, A. (2006) Acoustic parameters of dog barks carry emotional information for humans. *Applied Animal Behaviour Science* 100, 228–240.

Range, F., Viranyi, Z. and Huber, L. (2007) Selective imitation in domestic dogs. *Current Biology* 17, 868–872.

Range, F., Huber, L. and Heyes, C. (2011) Automatic imitation in dogs. *Proceedings of the Royal Society B* 278, 211–217.

RCVS (2012) *Code of Professional Conduct for Veterinary Surgeons*. RCVS, London.

Reichow, B., Barton, E.E., Good, L. and Wolcry, M. (2009) Brief Report: Effects of Pressure Vest Usage on Engagement and Problem Behaviors of a Young Child with Developmental Delays. *Journal of Autism and Developmental Disorders* 39(8), 1218–1221.

Romero, T., Konno, A. and Hasegawa, T. (2013) Familiarity bias and physiological responses in contagious yawning by dogs support link to empathy. PLoS ONE 8(8): e71365. Available at: http://www.plosone.org/article/info:doi/10.1371/journal.pone.0071365 (accessed 27 August 2013).

Rooney, N.J. and Cowan, S. (2011) Training methods and owner–dog interactions: links with dog behaviour and learning ability. *Applied Animal Behaviour Science* 132, 169–177.

Salman, M.D., New, J.G., Scarlett, J.M., Kris, P.H., Ruch-Gaille, R. and Hetts, S. (1998) Human and animal factors related to the relinquishment of dogs and cats in 12 selected animal shelters in the United States. *Journal of Applied Animal Welfare* 3, 207–226.

Schalke, E., Stichnoth, J., Ott, S. and Jones-Baade, R. (2007) Clinical signs caused by the use of electric training collars on dogs in everyday life situations. *Applied Animal Behaviour Science* 105, 369–380.

Schenkel, R. (1946) *Expression Studies on wolves: Captivity Observations*. Zoological Garden, Basle and the Zoological Institute of the University of Basle, Basle.

Schilder, M.B. and van der Borg, J.A.M. (2004) Training dogs with help of the shock collar: short and long term behavioural effects. *Applied Animal Behaviour Science* 85, 319–334.

Shepherd, K. (2002) Development of behaviour, social behaviour and communication in dogs. In: Horwitz, D., Mills, D. and Heath, S. (eds) *BSAVA Manual of Canine and Feline Behavioural Medicine*, 2nd edn. BSAVA, Gloucester, UK.

Shors, T.J. (2004) Learning during stressful times. *Learning and Memory* 11, 137–144.

Stead, A.C. (1982) Euthanasia in the dog and cat. *Journal of Small Animal Practice* 58, 37–43.

Stephenson, J. and Carter, M. (2009) The use of weighted vests with children with autism spectrum disorders and other disabilities. *Journal of Autism and Developmental Disorders* 39(1), 105–114.

Stevenson, D.D. and Kowalski, M.L. (2012) *Reactions to Aspirin and Other Non-steroidal Anti-inflammatory Drugs, An Issue of Immunology and Allergy Clinics*. Elsevier Health Sciences, Philadelphia, USA.

Topal, J., Gácsi, M., Miklósi, A., Viranyi, Z., Kubinyi, E. and Csányi, V. (2005) Attachment to humans: a comparative study on hand-reared wolves and differently socialized dog puppies. *Animal Behaviour* 70, 1367–1375.

Trut, L. (1999) Early canid domestication: the Farm-Fox Experiment. *American Scientist,* 87(2), 160. Available at: http://www.american-scientist.org/issues/num2/early-canid-domestication-the-farm-fox-experiment/1 (accessed 10 May 2013).

Van Honk, J., Peper, J.S. and Schutter, D.J.L.G. (2005) Testosterone reduces unconscious fear but not consciously experienced anxiety: implications for the disorders of fear and anxiety. *Biological Psychiatry* 58, 218–225.

Vollmer, P.J. (1977) Do mischievous dogs reveal their 'guilt'? *Veterinary Medicine, Small Animal Clinician* 72(6), 1002–1005.

Wells, D. (2001) The effectiveness of a citronella spray collar in reducing certain forms of barking in dogs. *Applied Animal Behaviour Science* 73, 299–309.

Wells, D.L. and Hepper, P.G. (2000) Prevalence of behaviour problems reported by owners of dogs purchased from an animal rescue shelter. *Applied Animal Behaviour Science* 69, 55–65.

Index